ATOMIC FITNESS

The Alternative to Drugs, Steroids, Wacky Diets, and Everything Else That's Failed

STEVE MICHALIK

MR. USA • MR. AMERICA • MR. UNIVERSE

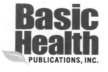

T0273405

The information contained in this book is based upon the research and personal and professional experiences of the author. It is not intended as a substitute for consulting with your physician or other healthcare provider. Any attempt to diagnose and treat an illness should be done under the direction of a healthcare professional.

The publisher does not advocate the use of any particular healthcare protocol but believes the information in this book should be available to the public. The publisher and author are not responsible for any adverse effects or consequences resulting from the use of the suggestions, preparations, or procedures discussed in this book. Should the reader have any questions concerning the appropriateness of any procedures or preparation mentioned, the author and the publisher strongly suggest consulting a professional healthcare advisor.

Basic Health Publications, Inc.
28812 Top of the World Drive
Laguna Beach, CA 92651
949-715-7327

Library of Congress Cataloging-in-Publication Data

Michalik, Steve.
    Atomic fitness : the alternative to drugs, steroids, wacky diets, and everything else that's failed / Steve Michalik.
        p. cm.
    Includes bibliographical references and index.
    ISBN-13: 978-1-59120-168-7
    ISBN-10: 1-59120-168-3
    1. Physical fitness. 2. Exercise. 3. Health. I. Title.

    RA781.M449   2006
    613.7'1—dc22

                                                        2006014284

Editor: Roberta W. Waddell
Photographers: Larry Tallis (exercise photos) and Denny (vintage photos)
Typesetting/Book design: Gary A. Rosenberg
Cover design: Mike Stromberg

Printed in the United States of America

10   9   8   7   6   5   4   3   2   1

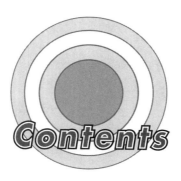

Contents

Appendices

Dedicated to . . .

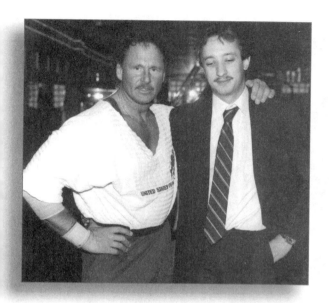

My brother Paul—
to whom I am
eternally grateful,
for without his wings
I would have never
flown again.

My Aussie rugby
mate, Joe Reaiche,
who pulled me from
the "demons of the
abyss" to regain
my true self.

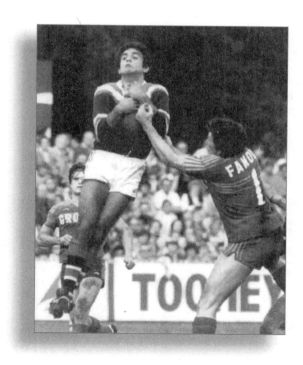

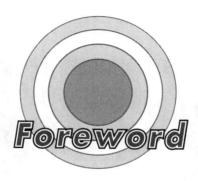

Foreword

A **CHAMPION** is one who visualizes a goal and goes after it with enough passion, knowledge, and desire to attain that goal. There are many champions. A **LEGEND** is one who becomes a champion and then uses that same passion, knowledge, and desire to help others attain their goals. There are few legends.

Steve Michalik is a LEGEND.

Steve has imbued in others the spirit, discipline, and knowledge necessary to enable them to become champions. His drive and commitment to help others is unparalleled. The book you now hold in your hands is a very powerful tool. It is the equivalent of a hammer to a carpenter. This information is essential in helping you attain your fitness and bodybuilding goals. Utilizing its principles of Atomic Fitness, or Intensity/Insanity, will enable you to reach goals you never thought were possible in bodybuilding. Millions of people exercise daily in hopes of reaching their goals. Few will ever achieve their goals because they lack the knowledge necessary to become successful. You wouldn't attempt to travel across the United States for the first time without consulting a good map to reach your destination. Steve's book is the map that will pinpoint your destination and your goals, chart the course, and guarantee your arrival. I have reached many of my destinations because I allowed Steve Michalik to be my navigator in my quest to reach my own bodybuilding and fitness goals. Steve's knowledge and commitment to excellence have also afforded me the ability to help thousands of others reach their fitness and bodybuilding goals. Read this book, absorb the information, and strive to be the best you can be. You cannot fail with Steve's direction to success!

—John DeFendis, Mr. USA

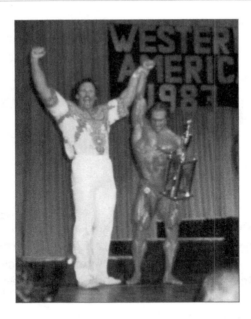

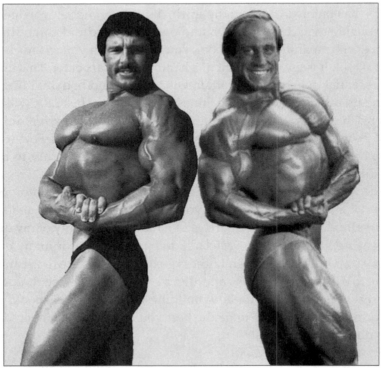

Two Champions—Two Legends: Steve Michalik and John DeFendis

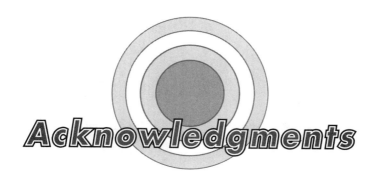

Acknowledgments

First, I would like to acknowledge myself for being able to accomplish what I have through the adversity and trauma of growing up in an emotionally abusive, dysfunctional, and suppressive household. Through my faith in the almighty and in myself, I was able to persevere and overcome. May this be a lesson of inspiration to all who feel helpless and hopeless.

I would next like to thank my partner and assistant, Darlene. Without her relentless and persistent support, neither I nor this book would be here today.

I would also like to acknowledge my wife, Tina, and my children, for believing in me.

My sincerest thanks go to Boris Mlawer and his son Ira who brought us together. Boris's experience and guidance throughout this project was priceless. Not only is he a consummate professional in all he pursues, but on a personal level, his genuine warmth and enthusiasm, coupled with intelligence and wisdom, led me to think of him as the father I longed to have.

I would like to extend thanks and recognition to my good friend Larry Tallis for the relentless hours and hours he put into creating the images for this book. Also, my thanks go out to my technical assistants Emy Bradley and Mike Manavian who were always up to the task.

I would also like to acknowledge Saul Katz for his wisdom and teaching throughout our friendship, which has made me a better man.

My sincerest gratitude goes to my publisher, Norman Goldfind, for taking a chance on me.

I would like to thank my spiritual mentor, Joe Reaiche, for helping to pull me out of the muck of life and showing me the light of freedom. And finally, I would like to acknowledge my successor and truest of all believers, John DeFendis, Mr. USA.

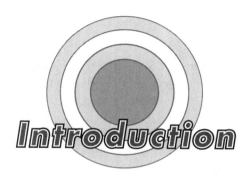

Introduction

I f you read everything there is to read on exercise and fitness, if you hire the best trainer money can buy, and even if you exercise at the best-equipped gym you can find, your results will still be merely ordinary.

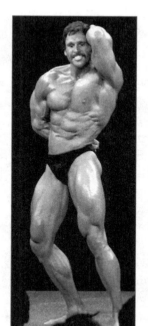

Gym memberships are up. Sales of books and videos on fitness are up. Information on diet and nutrition is abundant. There are more personal trainers now than ever, and yet there is 60 percent obesity in the United States. Heart disease is the number-one killer. Weak bones and soft muscles are the norm. Obviously, there is an epidemic of misinformation. The Atomic Fitness System will remove you from this maze of confusion. Ordinary is unacceptable, and only extraordinary will be tolerated.

IT'S HIGH TIME YOU DISCOVER THE TRUTH

I always get excited walking into a bookstore. The smell of new books and the colors and designs of the book covers stimulate my senses. During a typical visit, I asked a sales associate for the fitness and exercise section and was told to go three aisles down and then turn right. There, I was amazed at the seemingly endless rows of exercise books on everything from Pilates to water fitness, but what caught my interest most was the section on intense exercise—intense this, maximum intensity that. I thumbed through each book, laughing at the inaccuracies. Here were unknown authors, who have achieved little, or perhaps trained some athlete or celebrity, and now they're authorities. Trainers with barely enough knowledge to fit in an acorn are now preaching useless words of so-called wisdom. Each book has a little truth, surrounded by a lot of mumbo jumbo about the nature of intense training.

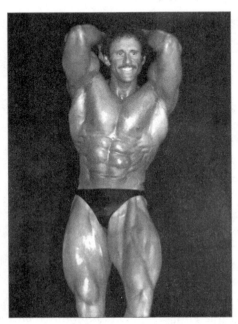

Ordinary is unacceptable.

One author claims to have developed the perfect *rep* (repetition). He says if you perform reps in a slow, controlled manner, it builds strength. Maybe, but it does little in the way of increasing the size or shape of the muscle, and it puts undue stress on the joints. I know because I did this workout a long time ago when Arthur Jones, of Nautilus fame, introduced it. I gave it a really good try until my joints started giving out and my neck and back were in constant stress, and still, there was no gain in muscle mass. My experience was no doubt duplicated by others because most people have abandoned this system. I have found that one of the limiting factors in exercise is an individual's strength, and believe me, you have to be strong to do those absurdly slow reps. So, I guess if you're willing to waste a year or two building the strength required for this system, it might work for you, especially if you have a good orthopedic surgeon. This *perfect-reps* author also says, "The strength system is ideal for any young athlete—children as young as ten can begin." Well, I don't know about you, but I don't want any ten-year-old doing this, or any weight training, until her or his bones have grown sufficiently, usually after puberty has set in. Another trainer says, and I quote, "To reduce the risk of injury, it is important for athletes to train both push and pull muscle groups." Well, Mr. Trainer, for your information, muscles only pull. They may give the illusion of pushing, but they don't.

I could go on and on. The truth is, you are bombarded by false information and misinformation. What dictates the truth is the ability to demonstrate your claim. The Atomic Fitness System has produced champions in every field of endeavor. It works. The only limiting factor is you and your ability to understand the facts. You drive the beast and the beast is you.

With the Atomic Fitness System, limitations no longer exist. This is true. Heredity need not be an obstacle, but only if you understand the interrelationship of the body and resistance. If you truly understand the body, the mind, and the method, then you will go a long way toward creating and building that fabulous body, and demonstrating the ultimate you. You must not repeat the errors of most who fail to recognize the benefits of the exercise method put forward in this book. For years, doctors (who, incidentally, die younger than most professionals) rejected the benefits of intense exercise, and suggested walking around the block a couple of times instead. Although such biases against this method of training still exist, years of proven results cannot be denied. Also, you don't need to obtain a degree in biophysics in order to understand and utilize the data.

THE ATOMIC FITNESS SYSTEM

Atomic Fitness, otherwise known as Atomic Intensity/Insanity or Atomic Force, refers to a group of fundamental principles of biology and physics that interact and function together as a whole in order to control energy, matter, space, and time. This is done with my unique exercise routines, knowledge of nutrition, and understanding of the workings of the inner mind. This Atomic Fitness System combines mental and physical movement with force, intelligence, and speed to bring about a biological change.

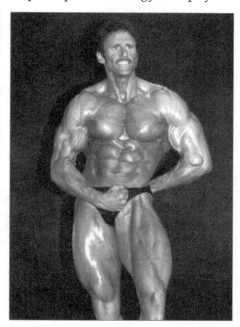

As used in this book, the word "atomic" relates to the amount of force put upon, and released in, the body to effect a physical change in an extremely short amount of time. As used here, time is a measurement of space. Shrink time and you collapse space, resulting in tremendous force, a force that has created

The more you know,
the more able you become.

the universe and has the ability to change it and everything in it, including the body. The reverse is also true—if you shrink space, you collapse time. These conditions bring about a significant change in matter—in this case, muscle and fat—and all the exercises and mental discipline in this book can create such a state.

In writing this book, I want to communicate to you what I know and what I've felt during my many successful years as a bodybuilder. And the term "bodybuilder" should be looked at as just that—an individual who wishes to build his or her body for whatever purpose.

Building a body is no different from how you would approach any other building project. You must first have a vision of what you want to build, of what exactly you are look-ing to do. Don't cheat yourself. Go for it all. Once you have determined your goal, be it health, appearance, or both, you'll have a starting point. Next, you'll need a blueprint, and that blueprint should show you exactly how to go about it. After that, you'll need some help in carry-ing out that blueprint. You'll need a skilled worker, someone you can trust, especially, with this particular building project—*you*.

The theories and principles set forth in this book work, and they work fast. What really determines how far you will get on your project is in the essence of each human being. There are those, like myself, who are relentless in their efforts,

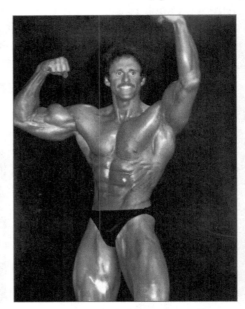

Only those who have been to the battle . . .

and then there are those who need guidance and understanding to get them through. Regardless of who you are and how you view life, this book will change the way you perceive your current state of reality. The sense of who you are and what you're doing becomes very clear as you embark on the journey of Atomic Fitness and see how it affects not only your body, but also your mind. Hidden in each of us are suppressed emotions and thoughts. Each of these hidden emotions (what I refer to as "mis-emotions") and thoughts were created by force, and the training principles in this book create tremendous body force, which unleashes those old suppressed body emotions. It sounds wild, but it works. Your body is just waiting for you to unleash all that stored negative energy.

It is, therefore, of the utmost importance that you fully understand how to train your body to obtain the greatest benefits. For starters, every time you do the Atomic Fitness routines, you need to block out all external thoughts and focus on your task. You will determine for yourself that it is necessary to work as hard as possible, and as you do this, you will feel excited and exhilarated, and enjoy a sense of freedom. You will be in a state of "cause," meaning you're in control. You will cause the outcome. This is freedom in its purest sense—a freedom seldom experienced elsewhere in life.

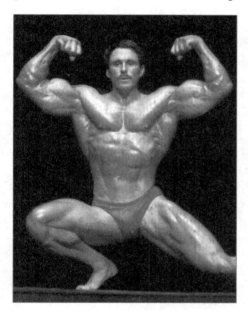

... can possibly understand the WAR!

During exercise, it is important to understand that it isn't how heavy a resistance is, it's how much force you can generate during that exercise, how much energy you can generate in each repetition—basically, how much mental force can you apply, and how much love, joy, and excitement you can put into the body as you move through the Atomic Fitness routines. You will learn to conquer and let go of fear. You will learn a lot about yourself and how tough you really are. And you know what? This knowledge of self will carry you through the rest of your life. These ideas of the mind and body are very powerful. As the ancients knew, these principles are at the core of existence.

I have traveled around the world and I have seen much, and what I have discovered is that all we believe to be reality is not. Once I unraveled this mystery through extensive study and meditation, I learned to know and perceive beyond the apparentness of reality. It all became crystal clear. Force created the universe and force will destroy it. All matter stems from force of some kind. The solution to all problems then stems from the use of energy and the force it creates, whether that force be intellectual, physical, or spiritual—the Atomic Fitness System integrates all three.

Physics teaches us that matter is held together by the forces, two forces being what is referred to as the strong force and the weak force. They pull at each other, creating stability. We use this secret of the universe to build bodies that are strong, look good, and last.

Thought is faster than light. Light is energy. Energy condensed is matter. Therefore, if you think it before it is apparent, it will be there waiting for you. I urge you to place your powers of thought into the body. Create positive images in your mind, and your body will follow that path.

Newton expressed his viewpoint of the universe as three-dimensional, with length, width, and depth. This, of course, applies to the human body. He explained that time, or duration, is merely a measuring device. Einstein expanded on this by explaining that dimensions are not consistent, and that time is variable. Simply put, duration of effort (in this case exercise) and speed of movement have a resounding effect upon the body. I use these principles in the Atomic Fitness System to bring about incredible results.

Much can be said about the science of the universe and how it ultimately affects lives, in this case, building a body—but that's a subject for another book entirely. For now, I have researched this data and come to the undeniable and demonstrated truth that the Atomic Fitness System works.

As you exercise, you should study the motion you're about to perform and determine how you can increase the force. For example, in any chest or shoulder press, as you lift the weight, force your hands inward. They do not move, but an isometric force (that is, a muscle contraction against resistance) is created while you move the resistance. For back work, the opposite

Facts You Should Have

■ The harder you do aerobics, the less fat you burn.

■ The longer you exercise, the less chance you have of getting in shape and building muscle.

■ You can't overtrain.

■ Fat doesn't make you fat.

■ Heavy weights don't build muscle.

■ Eating before a workout will *not* provide energy.

is true. You need to pull outward in an isometric effort. This will enhance the movement a hundredfold.

Remember, the velocity of the movement or exercise is of extreme importance. Einstein stated that, as velocity increases, time expands. This works beautifully in bodybuilding. Since the Atomic Fitness System increases intensity and incorporates the principle of velocity, it can be instantly seen how this applies to building a body quickly. What you want to do is create as much force on the muscle as possible, in the shortest period of time. Not only does the increased force directly impact the state of the muscle, but indirectly, you've created a greater period of recovery time for muscle growth. So basically, what I am stating here is that high-intensity exercise diminishes exercise time while expanding recovery time. If Einstein had only exercised, he would have been Mr. Olympia.

Two-minute butt, six-minute abs, eight-minute chest . . . If you're doing more, you're doing more than is needed, and accomplishing less. It's not time that builds a body, it's force. Reduce time and space, increase energy, and you will affect mass—mass in this case being fat and muscle. The Atomic Fitness System delivers fast, intense training principles that produce optimum results. It is the ultimate battle plan for defeating the "I have no time to exercise" idea. This state-of-the-art, scientific program conquers conventional wisdom with alternative breakthroughs. You now have an action plan that puts it all together for you.

The Atomic Fitness System combines the very best advancements in modern thinking with the wisdom of the great minds of the past. It is supported by years of research and decades of results. It roots out the false data and propaganda associated with exercise. It wipes out conventional exercise methods that are time-consuming and harmful. Research has come a long, long way, and the Atomic Fitness System is packed with life-changing information that makes it possible to alter your physique in the shortest time possible. I will give you the facts that will allow you to win the battle for your body. You no longer need to feel overwhelmed. You deserve every chance to achieve your goals. The Atomic Fitness System delivers hope beyond hope. From your first workout, you'll restore energy, vitality, a sense of self, and a renewed confidence that you can accomplish all you desire.

HOW TO USE THIS BOOK

The following chapters are designed to bring an awareness of the facts and provide clear instructions on how to apply the principles presented. I have attempted, in as simple a manner as possible, to outline the points of knowledge necessary for producing ultimate results.

Part One of this book lays out my personally developed theories and explains the origins of such intriguing methods as the Intensity/Insanity system of building muscles. These easy-to-understand exercises start with preconditioning routines to provide a foundation of optimum fitness levels in order to prepare you for the real work to follow. From there, the routines progress from beginning, intermediate, and advanced, to super-advanced routines. Sections on abdominals, hips, and butt are also included.

Part Two takes up the body's basic anatomy and explores the role of nutrition. This is followed by a selection of recipes designed to provide maximum benefits to the body. Testimonials, a glossary, appendixes, references, and a full index are also provided toward the end of the book.

It has long been understood that exercise is capable of producing significant increases in strength and clarity of mind. Even prehistoric humans appeared to understand this, as early archeological finds show evidence of humans engaging in exercise and conditioning. Today's society requires men and women to strive for perfection and unheard-of levels of fitness and skill. My goal is simple—to educate you in the ways that can bring about such dynamic change in your thinking that you will never be the same again.

Looking into the future, you can see your final goals being realized. Now you must do it. Teaching old dogs new tricks may be difficult, but it is not impossible. Although much bias and rumor plague society, you must not be afraid to challenge current beliefs and see the light of the new. For all that is new is as old as the creation of the body itself. The principles I have brought forth are new only to a point of present understanding. The body and mind work in a certain way. The mind follows exact rules of behavior, regardless of your intentions. You must conquer with understanding what seemed unconquerable in the past. You must come to discover and live a new reality. You must have a love of life so profound that you become one with all. Be responsible to yourself, seek truth, and knowledge will follow. Then and only then will you finally be *in control.*

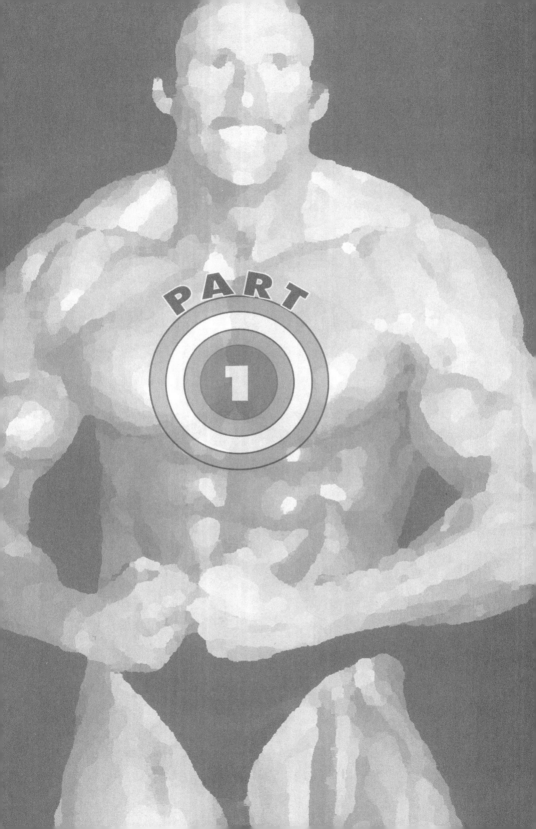

PART

1

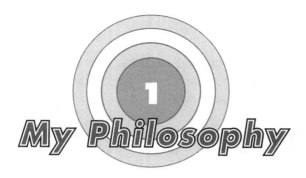

My Philosophy

The initial section of this book provides valuable insight into my philosophy regarding life and the principles of Atomic Fitness, as well as why it works and how to apply it.

In your quest for physical perfection, it's important to know who and what you are. Are you a body or an incredible being? Are you more than a mere animal? Who are you really? The one thing you know for certain is that you are somewhere. Therefore, you know you're in this game and it's called life. What you should know is that your every waking hour is spent trapped in a body and imprisoned by a mind. It is difficult to comprehend this scenario, let alone figure it out. To figure it out, you must know the truth. What is the truth? What is the reality? There are many realities, but only one real truth. The truth is, you are a being living symbiotically with a body. You want it to change. It doesn't. Your power over this body will determine your success in all you seek to do. With that said, let me relay what I have seen and experienced as the truth.

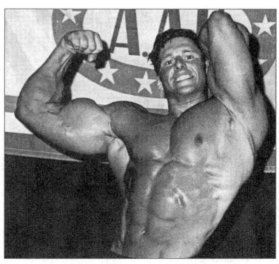

A strong mind + a strong body = absolute success and total supremacy.

Many millions of words have been written about life and its purpose. They cover all bases and viewpoints—physiological, psychological, and philosophical. It is my belief that less than 5 percent of this information comes close to any workable knowledge. Therefore, the bulk of this book is devoted to bringing forth an understanding and correcting that which is misunderstood. Welcome to the journey. I can assure you it's a fascinating one. My mission is simple, to provide the basic information needed to produce a better you. The more you know, the more capable you become. This is true in exercise and in life itself. People have asked me, why write this book? With its different approach to the physiology, philosophy, and psychology of building a body, it is certain to stir up controversy. My response is simple: It is worth anything I may encounter to reveal the truth as I have come to understand it. Nothing in this universe is new. All that is to be known has already been discovered. The trick is to see through all the muck, confusion, and false data so that what is valuable may be revealed and recorded.

After decades of observation, data collection, and application, I felt it was time to present my findings to the world. This technology, this data, this truth, should not be lost. Confusion and controversy should be put to rest. This data need not be boring or complicated. It should be rapidly assimilated and applied. True understanding of the information should expose a mountain of false data associated with the game of life. Life is a game. Building a body is a game. You can't win any game unless you know what you're up against. What you don't know will kill you in ways you can't even imagine. Fear, failure, and frustration are all part of not knowing. So, to those who would

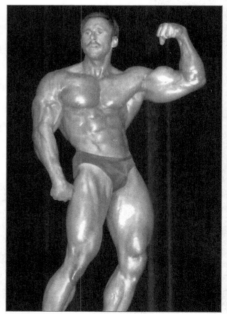

Know who you are.

disgrace this majestic field of endeavor with false hope, malice, ignorance, and misinformation, let them be exposed for who and what they are. I put forth that a life based on seeking the truth will always surpass one based on a lie.

I wish to thank all those in the past and present who have worked without notoriety or reward so that others may play this valiant game. The original objective of this game of life is simple: to survive and out-create life. This still remains life's purpose today, and continues to elude all those who have played. Society's most established masterminds have only managed to collide with the task, reaching conclusions that seem to provide further diluted data and invoking more unwarranted confusion. Man has doomed himself by the inability to know, relying entirely on what he is told to think and believe. There lies the problem. Man rarely questions and is clueless about the intention of the game, which is to bring about his demise.

The best teachers of every era have yet to create players who can win and produce solutions consistently. You can only wonder at the variety of *almosts* and *could-have-beens* that cover this glorious planet. People look to gurus to somehow magically open the gates to the secrets of life and happiness, but unfortunately, they've proven they're still not up to the task.

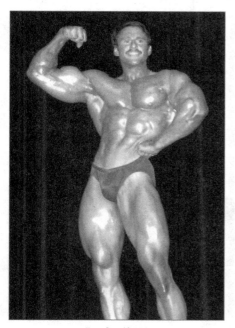

Perfection.

This meek standard that has been presented is coming to an end. The creation of a new era of awakening is at hand. Those who venture to learn the truth will survive. Those who do not are doomed to be earth zombies. Those who can confront life will live, and that is all that is asked.

As you may have noticed, I put strong emphasis on the development of the mind, for the underdeveloped mind will be your barrier to success. It would be pointless to teach you the aspects of building the ultimate body through exercise without devoting equal time to the ultimate mind. Whichever one is weaker is the one that will hold you back, keep you down, and prevent you from moving forward.

The human mind is engaged in perceiving and remembering data, resolving problems, and understanding conclusions. The ability to receive and retain information that leads to conclusions and problem solving is directly related to overcoming the noise of misinformation that vibrates in

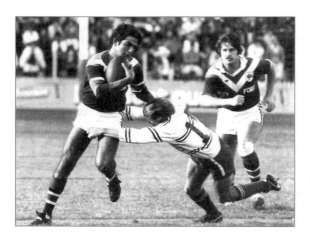

Mental force is the manifestation of emotion. Physical force is the manifestation of motion.

your head. This vibration is the ultimate penalty for the body's involvement in the mind's affairs. The body has been designed with the postulate to survive. The body has a mind of its own that reacts to situations in the environment. This is not you. The mind you use is analytical. The mind the body uses usually results in stupidity, aberration, and eventual pain. Those who concede control to this body mind will eventually have less and less analytical control over the environment and their bodies, lowering their potential to succeed. Taking control and using your mind, pushing through barriers, overcoming obstacles, and disagreeing with failure raises your ability and intelligence, and thus moves you toward success. Both ability and intel-

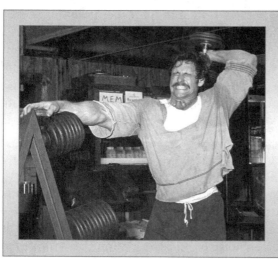

Levels of Force

Only through force can you conquer and win in this universe.

EFFORT—A lot of work, little gain.

EMOTION—A lot of mental stress, little gain.

SELF—Total certainty, endless gains.

ligence are necessary to persist. A highly developed body has force and power. A highly developed mind has knowingness and intelligence. Thus, a strong mind and a strong body equal absolute success and total supremacy. I can't state this enough.

Whatever your goal in life, whether it's to have a world-class physique, or to obtain your own personal fitness goals, it is a game, as all of life is a game. The body and the mind are two players in this game. Sometimes they work together, sometimes they oppose each other. The body will oppose vigorously any change made to its structure. Only through the force and the power of the mind can you overcome this resistance. *You are your weakest link!*

This mind game is an adventure. It is the ultimate game, and it will determine your future successes and failures. Even a little understanding of how it works will give you a great advantage over others. In this book, I discuss a few subjects that I feel relate to your success. Much exists on the subject of the mind and its control over your everyday behavior. Perhaps someday you will want to learn more about how the mind works and its relationship to you and your body. For now, the information provided here will put you miles ahead of everyone else and take your game to a level you never imagined.

As mentioned before, you are as strong as your weakest link. That link is the misinformation about what you are. Simply put, you are not a body, you are not a mind or brain, you are

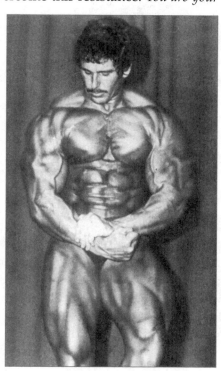

It's a battle between YOU and your BODY. I pray you win.

simply you. You occupy a body that uses a brain and its software—the mind. When you exercise, the body wants you to fail. It will try to convince you to quit. It will try to enlist the brain to help make you fail. These are the voices in your head. They are not you. They are the voices of the cells attempting to revolt against any structural change made to the body due to exercise. The body will try to get you to decide you've had enough. This battle of wills pits you against your body, which is basically lazy and also frightened. It is programmed to resist any effort to change. Exercise, especially intense exercise, is designed to change your physical structure. To the body, this change is *non-survival*. The only way you can change a muscle is to create a non-survival environment in that muscle. This will instantly create that noise in your head telling you to quit. That noise is your enemy, and it will be your downfall if you allow it to be. You must conquer it, or it will most definitely conquer you.

Life is a GAME. The game I chose was BODYBUILDING.

A bodybuilder's mental attitude is extremely important. You must will your muscles to grow. You must hypnotize yourself into believing that anything is possible.

An important part of the Atomic Fitness System involves the use of voice recordings. You should make a tape, in your own voice, telling yourself that nothing is impossible, and describing yourself as you wish to be. Speak to yourself in a commanding voice and describe your ultimate physique in great detail. If you have a weak body part, enforce its growth potential to yourself. Think and speak only positives. Do not be afraid to love yourself and what you want to become. Never, ever, allow yourself a moment of self-doubt. You must firmly believe you will become all you desire. Place the finished tape at your bedside and play it at night, over and over, then once again before you train. If you dream it, you can become it, and one dream is worth a thousand realities. Thought is senior to matter (the human body). Whatever you put into the future, and hold to be true, you will become. Whatever you hold out in front of you, you will reach. Nothing, my friend, is impossible if you believe.

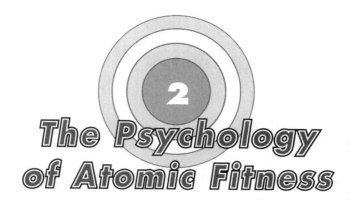

The Psychology of Atomic Fitness

There is this phenomenon called mind noise—those little voices that talk to you. Everyone has them, but no one talks about them, for it is difficult to acknowledge and confront these phenomena. It's neither the old story of devil versus angel or your conscience, it's the somatic—or body—mind, that is, all the cells in the body communicating through your mind, verbalizing viewpoints on survival, based on past experiences. These viewpoints are not necessarily in your greatest interest. They are intended to be good for the body. But you are not a body; you are you. You occupy a body in a form of symbiotic partnership, except it is most likely proportioned 90 percent to 10 percent in favor of your body, and you need to change that.

This chapter outlines various viewpoints and ideas about the mind. You will need to know and understand these viewpoints in order to progress through the Atomic Fitness System. They include the following:

- **The Psychology of You** discusses the game of life and how it applies to exercise and you.

- **The Psychology of Ability and Physical Change** discusses the mind/body slump and how it affects your mental and physical ability to produce change.

- **Life Is Energy** discusses the mind's energy and how to channel it toward your goals.

- **Technique to Eliminate Mind Noise** provides a method of taking back control of self.

THE PSYCHOLOGY OF YOU

Before you can know who and what you are, you must first understand what you've gotten yourself into.

In the beginning there was a cause, and that cause was to create a game. This has been true since the beginning of time and remains true today. In this case, the game is building a body.

In this game, some people believe intelligence is a substitute for experience. Others believe experience is senior to intelligence. None of this matters if you're not willing to observe the obvious and ignore the ranting of bias and rumor, the hearsay and naysayers. If you do this, you will discover the true path to physical perfection.

Building bodies has been around since the beginning of time. The ancients believed it godly to have physical perfection. Yet, from generation to generation, people have allowed themselves to get frustrated by their inability to achieve this ideal. They have allowed frustration to interfere with their goals of getting in shape and achieving their goals. It is a difficult enough game for anyone to master while being fully conscious, but nearly impossible for those in the state of unconsciousness that permeates today's society. We are constantly bombarded with false data from Madison Avenue and Hollywood. Such false data corrupts our ability to see the truth, placing us in a hypnotic state and preventing us from being able to absorb correct data.

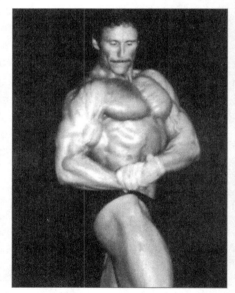

The way out is the way through, there is no way around. You must be willing to play to get through. Be "cause over life" . . . create.

No other endeavor presents its participants with as grand a purpose as the game of life. And no other purpose is more worthwhile than the pursuit of physical perfection. This game offers a passion that commences at birth and ends with death. It is not biased for either success or failure. It is encompassed by the vast landscapes set in nature's astounding creation, Earth. This game can provide a lifetime full of enjoyment or unbearable sorrow. Your purpose transcends all other games just by mere design. It requires assembling ideas, intelligence, honor, integrity, and perseverance. It pits knowledge against power, yet asks you to combine the two. It asks you to move forward with a sense of the unknown, while demanding performance at the highest levels over the period of an entire life, in an environment that can range from desert heat to frigid chill.

At the same time, it is creating the ultimate test of tests. This test mentally challenges the quest to attain perfection, while bombarding its participants with the fiercest distractions and most tempting passions of life. Now *this* is a game—a balanced game that equally tests the mind's ability to focus, the body's rudiments, and the true sense of what and who you are. Building a body through exercise is a passion, a true purpose that tests the mind and spirit.

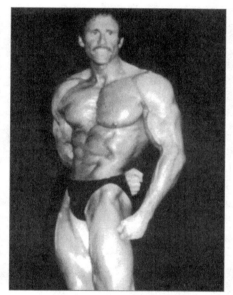

The ability to change physically lies completely with you.

This game offers no guarantee for success, no multimillion-dollar compensation packages for injuries, or bench time. What's required is to show up and do your best. You're in complete control of the outcome. There are no real opponents other than self. You are friend and enemy. Everyone starts out equally with those they battle, and through their own efforts, their fate is determined.

Life is a game of integrity, honor, and tradition, the rules of which are self-imposed and self-enforced. The game is you and your body, a game you must win. I will show you how.

THE PSYCHOLOGY OF ABILITY AND PHYSICAL CHANGE

The loss of ability, as well as the inability to physically change, is due to a condition known as the mind/body slump. What is this? Simply put, it is a metabolic condition where the mind and body are working at less than optimal levels and against each other. This condition, also known as the somatic mind conflict, occurs when the analytical mind seems to shut off and the body runs on automatic. In this state, the mind ceases to create. It runs on past experiences and cannot contemplate present or future conditions. This is a less than desirable situation. If you think you're in control of your body, try to will a cut to stop bleeding. Try to hold your breath for more than a minute. If you have a cold, make it go away. If you have a toothache, stop the pain. If you happen to develop an incurable disease, decide to overcome it. If you're unable to do any of these things, I guess you'll decide you're not in control of much in your body except, perhaps, blowing your nose.

There was, however, a time when at mankind's purest, people had a complete and total command over the body. They dealt with present and future considerations to effect change. However, through time and evolution, this ability was lost. The human mind today is subservient to the will of the somatic mind (or body). Today's mind runs on machinery and circuits, reacting to, rather than causing, change. It is very difficult to produce a positive physical change in a body that is designed to resist change. This is one of life's greatest illusions. People believe they're in control, when they are actually being controlled by a biochemical condition known as emotion and somatic thought. This brings me to the main reason people fail to create physical change.

The limiting factor in building muscle tissue, and performing exercise to its maximum, is what I call *mis-emotion*. When in a state of mis-emotion, known as a mind slump, there is an inability to demonstrate skills, including those necessary for exercise. Tasks seem hard to accomplish; things just don't seem to go right. You may feel tired and drained, or lose your drive and ambition. When this biochemical condition occurs, you believe it is you. It's not. You're in a mind slump, a condition in which hormones and the nervous system dictate your emotions and moods and may prevent you from reaching your full potential. You've also gotten into a state in which your liver is too tired and toxic to provide energy relief. In order to build a body quickly and achieve maximum benefits, you need to be in full control of your body. *With the use of the Atomic Fitness techniques featured in this book, you will learn how to control your body to overcome this biochemical condition.*

Basically, the body is a machine. The system's organs and cells are simply part of the body's machinery. This machine can be run on automatic, or it can be controlled through the use of your mind. The body controlled by you is at your command, thereby allowing you access to the full range of abilities and skills necessary to build your body. When you're out of the slump condition, you're basically in the driver's seat of life. You're in control, making all the right decisions, all the correct turns, and absorbing all that life can offer.

This is a far better way to play the game than being in the mind slump, living your life on automatic and allowing decisions and actions to be based on data previously collected and stored by the body. These automatic mechanisms may not be life positive. They may include upsets, urges, habits, and dysfunctional thoughts, all of which interfere with analytical thought and create an inability to achieve your goals. All of this plays back to you during your workout sessions and can cause you to question your willing-

ness to continue with that workout. Remember, you can only make effective decisions when they are based on accurate perceptions. Therefore, you need to quiet mis-emotions in the body and let the mind's energy flow. This energy will build a strong body, paving the way for optimal health and training. Failure will become less likely and weaknesses less severe. When the body and mind work efficiently, there is a great sense of command over life. Ability to perform increases, body structure changes, fat loss and muscle tone happen naturally, purposes and goals soar, and strength is a given, as weakness and fatigue become things of the past.

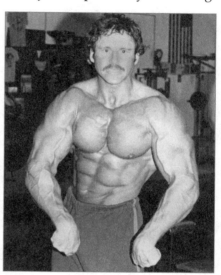

Tolerance and patience are signs of strength. Embrace the barriers.

How then do we stay out of the mind slump? This question has been asked for centuries. Wise men, scientists, doctors, athletes, religious leaders, and society in general have all searched the ends of the earth for a solution. The answer is actually quite simple. Life is a constant balance of many factors, including energy and matter, force and intelligence, power and knowledge. There is also a state of supreme balance between the body and the mind that pushes all else aside. Clearing a path through the maze of confusion and frustration, there is only one way to escape the slump, and that is on the back of physical and mental power. To take back the power of your mind, you must balance the body's chemistry with the energy of the mind. When you do this, you quiet the noise of mis-emotion in your head. Life becomes more observable, enabling greater levels of concentration and the full use of your senses. You will push forward to the ultimate experience. You will perceive life fully and train with incredible force and power.

It's important to remember that you can't observe what you can't perceive, and you can't perceive the optimum benefit from your training unless you're fully there to mentally observe what is going on. An unconditioned body has to work harder to accomplish basic tasks. An unconditioned mind has to process more useless information that is filtered through the body. A body with chemistry that is out of balance due to poor conditioning will be very noisy. This constant noise interferes with the decision-making process, creating body circuits that negatively influence your ability to think, making true concentration during exercise impossible. It's similar to a car that's out of tune. The engine will be noisy and the car will not run at maximum efficiency. When a car is tuned up, however, you can hardly hear the engine and you can have confidence in its performance. The human body is the same way. Fine-tune it, and it will run quietly and perform incredibly. Putting the body in harmony allows you to operate fully and with certainty. Muscle fatigue and failure become unacceptable. The voices of doubt in your head will be replaced with clarity. The Atomic Fitness method of training will increase endurance and stamina, while allowing you to relax and achieve calmness within your mind.

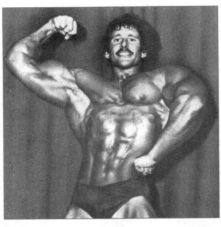

Personal integrity is your shield against that which stands between you and success. Be brave!

How does physical and mental condition affect performance and the ability to exercise? They relate to each other in several ways. A strong mental and physical condition enhances exercise. Ability, performance, and the process of burning fat and building muscle depend on several factors, all greatly influenced by exercise. These factors are metabolism, flexibility, muscle size, muscle tone, speed, stamina, strength, and the ability to resist injury. Add these up and you have an individual's total ability to change the body. The ability to perform a skill, in this case exercise, depends on the ability to create force and the willingness to use it. Training ability is influenced by the development of the factors listed above. An individual must be totally in the present during exercise in order to achieve full concentration.

Simply put, if you're not fully there, you can't concentrate. If your mind is elsewhere, your body will run on automatic and simply try to survive; its idea of survival will be to get you to fail, thereby eliminating any perceived threat. That is why it is necessary to have total control and certainty over your mental condition. This is an absolute necessity for building a physique or developing a skill, and it is truly the secret of the Atomic Fitness System. If mastered, you will see results happen so fast they will rock your reality and make you question your sanity.

Everyone is born with one or more of the factors listed above. It is the goal of Atomic Fitness to bring as many of these factors into balance as possible. This is what brings about success. The individual who can come close to balancing all these factors will have the talent necessary to achieve his or her goal; the higher the degree of balance, the greater the talent to succeed.

> Talent is the ability to focus on the task before you. It is the ability to perceive and duplicate without distortion, and then demonstrate it. Training requires talent, the key for the doorway into a dimension where all is possible.

LIFE IS ENERGY

Life is energy. Life consumes energy. All matter is made of energy. It stands to reason that you should learn how to control the energy that runs the mind, the body, and life. The Atomic Fitness System will teach you how.

You must be in total control of energy to achieve your goal. Mind energy—the energy the mind both creates and uses—is the most powerful force in the universe. It is vast and limitless. This force knows no boundaries; it makes no moral judgments; it does not differentiate between good or bad, friendly or evil. You can utilize the mind's energy for production or destruction. The Atomic Fitness System utilizes the mind's energy to create physical change in the body.

▶ Step 1

Keep your integrity. This is a state of unbroken wholeness. It is a condition of not being marred or violated, of being unimpaired and uncorrupted, of maintaining a soundness. It is a condition of moral principle and character, of truth and untainted virtue, even in the face of adversity. It's important to engage life with self-confidence. Never back down from your purpose.

Never allow yourself to feel hopeless or demoralized. These emotions use up lots of energy, and this negative energy will permeate your cells and mind. Stay strong. Fight off mis-emotion and keep your ethics and morals high. Maintain your integrity and you will never feel the effect of negative energy. With this outlook, you will never quit or abandon your purpose, whether it is health, strength, or a championship physique.

▶ Step 2

Leave all negative action in the past. Always look at your life as a new unit of time. Calm your mind and refuse to own any negative thoughts. Save your energy for solutions, not problems. Tolerance and patience are signs of strength. The difficult times, the barriers you just can't seem to get past, provide the best opportunity for gaining useful experience and developing inner strength.

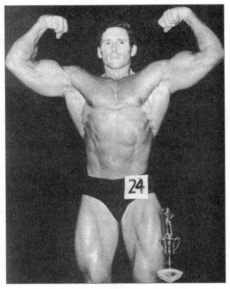

"Steve, you'll never be anything."
Yeah, RIGHT!

In your training, you will come across barriers. These are good. It is strange but true, a barrier is a brother to success. Every time you run into some life barrier, if you persist and don't back down (remember integrity), you will beat the barrier and play with much more vigor and success. You will learn and grow. You will be tested. After all, life is a game. And what is a game? It is play versus stops. It is success versus barriers. It is *I want* versus *No you can't.* The secret is—you *can.* If you persist, believe in yourself, stay in the now, and maintain integrity, you will win. Every time you win the mind war, you get stronger. Most, on some level, quit and fail the test. This will not be you. The game is set up to make you fail; otherwise, there would be no game. A win-win scenario is not a game. It's boring and the participants soon lose interest. So embrace the losses. For it's win some, lose some that keeps the game going. Think about it. Isn't all of life like this? No barrier, no game. You can reach your goal. There are no setbacks, no failures, only learning experiences.

Again, don't be upset over a loss or a barrier. Barriers create space and time. Space and time give you a chance to evaluate and decide the next course of action. Embrace the barriers. If the barriers were removed, people would eventually run out of space and then run out of time. Isn't this what happened to Elvis Presley? No more game, so he checked out. He simply ran out of things to do. He had no barrier left to overcome, so he became a victim of space and time. Relish the stops and bring them on. The wins become bigger. Your successes become greater. How many times have you seen a man retire from his job and his work challenges only to die shortly afterward? He simply ran out of play. No play, no life, no time. So bring on the hazards. Go right at them, and you know what? You'll live longer.

TECHNIQUE TO ELIMINATE MIND NOISE

The purpose of the following technique is to help you increase personal integrity so you can maintain a "here and nowness," along with the ability to conquer the voices of doom in your mind. It is this wall of voices that prevents you from training as hard as you really can and keeps you from achieving your goals.

Transgressions from your past have an adverse effect on your life now and on building the ultimate body in the present time. The goal is to uncover these transgressions. What you hope to achieve is an increased gain in personal integrity—a condition, or state, of no longer being divided against yourself, thus being whole and fully in the present. A position of integrity is a condition of power from which all else radiates.

Here Is How It Is Done

Read, and answer completely, the seventeen questions listed below. For each question, ask a subset of five questions (A through E as follows), until you've thoroughly completed each of the seventeen main questions and have reached the bottom of the list. At that point, start over again from the top, finding new answers. Keep cycling through the list until you eventually run out of answers. When you've done this, you will have silenced the mind noise that can interfere with your ability to play life's games. Use a separate piece of paper for your answers.

As an example, take the first question, "Have you ever denied yourself an opportunity?" Answer the question in the following five ways:

A. Who? B. What? C. Where? D. When? E. How was it a transgression?

Then write down any cognition (awareness) you may have after answering these questions, and how you feel about the transgression now. In the above case, an example would be as follows:

A. Me.

B. I didn't go to college because my father wanted me to work in his bakery.

C. In Chicago, in the town of Bayville, in my father's bakery.

D. When I was eighteen (June 11, 1976).

E. I wanted to go to college to become a teacher, but against my own knowingness, I worked in my father's bakery.

Cognition: I realized I am ultimately responsible for my actions and should have gone to college at any cost of hardship or loss.

Here are the seventeen integrity questions. Answer each as outlined in the example above. Go through the list as many times as necessary until you run out of answers.

1. Have you ever denied yourself an opportunity?

2. Is there something you won't let yourself have?

3. Have you ever deliberately made someone think badly of you?

4. Have you ever made someone punish you?

5. Have you ever distrusted yourself?

6. Have you ever made yourself sick?

7. Have you ever hurt yourself?

8. Is there something you haven't let yourself do?

9. Have you ever thought something was much too good for you?

10. Is there something you thought you didn't deserve?

11. Have you ever prevented yourself from accomplishments?

12. Is there something you won't let yourself feel?

13. Is there something you won't let yourself think?

14. Is there something you won't let yourself understand?

15. Is there something you won't let yourself know?

16. Is there something you won't let yourself create?

17. Have you ever betrayed yourself?

Every time you violate what you know, or do what you know you shouldn't, you build negative energy in the subconscious. And this negative energy will exert its influence on you every time you try to achieve a goal, in this case, exercising to your maximum potential.

DID YOU KNOW?
Helpful Hints and Tidbits to Help You Overcome the Psychological Barriers of Training

1. Thought travels faster than light, and light allows you to perceive your reality. So if you think it, and believe it, and make it your reality, it will be there waiting for you.

2. You are not a body. You simply occupy a body and use it to be mobile.

3. Pain originates in the brain and manifests in the area contacted. Overcome the origin and conquer the pain.

4. The mind is constructed of mental mass and energy that has been made by you to do work for you.

5. People consist of multiple cells that are seeking to survive and only survive.

6. The body is basically a machine. It follows basic rules of survival. It is necessary to understand these rules so you can break them.

7. Muscle memory is a recording of the physical universe where muscle action has taken place. It records time, place, and event.

8. A mental-image picture, or mock-up, of the way you wish to be or look is essential to any real progress. It is a copy of what you want to be. Create it, see it, become it.

9. A positive viewpoint is absolutely necessary for achieving your goal. The viewpoint is your awareness through which you can perceive your final goal.

10. An alternate personality is the identity of someone or something other than oneself that is assumed in order to accomplish a task. For example, the identity of a cook would not do well for a bricklayer. Nor would the identity of a procrastinator produce a bodybuilder or someone who is physically fit. Therefore, it is important to know who you are and to avoid alternate personalities that may interfere with your goals.

11. In order to be something, you must do something.

12. Everything is contained in some space. If you wish to be in great shape, or possess the body you desire, you must have an affinity for that space and be willing to occupy it. In other words, love yourself.

13. If you truly wish to make your dreams real, you must communicate with that dream, thereby bringing you to totally understand what it will take.

14. You were born to do great things. Don't fail yourself.

15. Wisdom is the most important thing on Earth.

16. Fear is a nonconfrontation of something in life. You can conquer anything you can confront.

17. You were created to cause an effect. Purposes cause effects.

18. Those who would stop you cannot confront your courage and desires, for it reminds them of their failures.

19. If they are to be achieved, your dreams must be believed, pursued, and always protected.

20. Your purpose must be born within you, not borrowed from another.

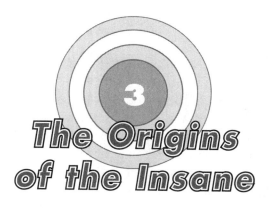

The Origins
of the Insane

"Steve! Steve! You're not going to believe what I have," cried a voice just outside my office at the gym. "Okay, Mikey, what now?" I replied to the excited figure, now standing beside me. What Mikey had was a copy of a book. I gazed at the cover, which read, *The Greatest Sports Stories of the Century*, and turning the pages, I noticed stories about Muhammad Ali, Secretariat, Barry Bonds, and other sport legends. When I reached the section Mikey had marked, there was the name Steve Michalik. It was *my* story. Me, Steve Michalik, among the greatest sports stories of all time! As I read the story in amazement, my mind flashed back to a time long ago that was not so amazing. . . .

It was cold, dark, and lonely in the closet that night, especially for a ten-year-old, but not too different from any other night when my dad decided I needed to be taught a lesson. Yet something *was* different this time, and it had nothing to do with the fact that I had stopped crying when he hit me with his belt, or that I no longer protested being thrown in the closet. It was me. I was different. The change had started just two nights before, after once again being cast into the abyss of that closet and suddenly noticing a stack of old comic books piled in the corner.

With all the courage I could muster, I ever so slowly opened the prison door of the closet just enough to let some light in. My heart pounded in my chest, and I hoped desperately that no noise would come from the door. It was silent. I was safe, for now anyway. I took a long, deep breath, settled down on the floor with my back against the closet wall, and started on the stack that would become the turning point of my life.

As I went through the stack, I could feel my heart pounding again, but this time it was from excitement. What lay before me was amazing. I was so captivated, my mind spun with thoughts of adventure, freedom, and yes, oh yes, power and strength. Ironically, there in the hell I'd been sentenced to, I found my inspiration. Courage, honesty, integrity, and loyalty to his country were all part of the creed of this comic book hero I'd stumbled across. For as long as I could remember, these had been the ideals I had aspired to, but all I had ever experienced was criticism, invalidation, and abuse. Not now. Not anymore. For now I had an ally—a role model. There was finally someone I could look up to. I would be like him. Even better, I decided nothing would stop me, and I would *become* . . . Captain America.

Each punishment night in my hideaway, I would read the adventures of Captain America, and marvel at how he would overcome injustices with his power and strength, intimidating others with his incredible physique. This was my solution to the tyranny I suffered at the hands of my father and brother. I concluded that wild dreams of revenge and justice were not enough. I needed a plan that would forever seal my fate, and the fate of anyone who attempted to get in my way.

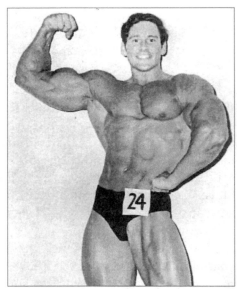

Steve Michalik, one of the youngest Mr. Americas.

Pondering this, it was soon clear that I knew nothing about how to be strong, and knew even less about my body or how to change it. But that, too, was about to change, as the fates, once again, stepped in.

I had contracted mumps and the family doctor made a house call to check me over (in those days, doctors made house calls). Dr. Merkin was an odd sort of man, short, stocky, and not particularly easy to look at. But he was kind and soft-spoken, welcome attributes considering my family circumstances. He was also inclined to talk a lot, a condition I intended to exploit.

I realized that kindly Dr. Merkin would know the human body and how it worked, but how would I convince him to help me in my quest to become strong and powerful? I called on the expertise of Captain America. What would he do? Be straightforward and honest, an inner voice cried out. Yes, I would just tell him my dream and he would understand.

"So, Mr. Michalik," he said after I blurted out my endgame, "you want to be Captain America . . . think you'd look good in those blue tights?"

"Not now, doctor, but maybe someday," I replied. He asked specifically what I wanted and I told him it wasn't what I wanted, it's what I needed—information about the body. "I need to know how it works, how bone and muscle grow."

"I think I have just what you need," Dr. Merkin replied. "Come to my office after hours, around six." The office was in his home just down the block from my house, a small home for a doctor, I thought, but this was the kind of man he was. I approached his door with great anticipation, and I can remember walking down the stairs to his office and gazing with amazement at all the books lining the walls—books filled with information about the human body. This was the storehouse of information I needed to succeed, and I was convinced that I was on the right path.

Dr. Merkin, who turned out to be very interested in helping me, handed me some muscle magazines. On the cover of one was a bodybuilder named Steve Reeves, a real live Captain America. At that point, I realized, with great disappointment, that if he was Captain America, I could never have that name. I also realized, though, that, just as Steve Reeves had done, I could conquer all my fears by being Mr. America. I decided to make that my goal. For the rest of my life, I would do whatever it took to become Mr. America.

Soon after this came my eleventh birthday, and like any other birthday, it went uncelebrated. However, these things weren't important anymore. The only thing that mattered was obtaining all the knowledge necessary to be a bodybuilding champion.

Reading the doctor's magazines that he had allowed me to take home gave me great insight into the world of bodybuilding. Seeing how others like me were able to achieve greatness and self-confidence through bodybuilding fueled my enthusiasm. Unfortunately, my father did not share my viewpoint. When he discovered me reading a muscle magazine he became furious. He told me that looking at pictures of men in magazines was disgraceful, and that I was nothing but a piece of garbage. I knew then I was on the right track. After all, anything my father disagreed with had to be right.

On my next visit to Dr. Merkin, I discussed what had happened. He was outraged and vowed to help with whatever I needed. It was the beginning of a fantastic journey. The following weeks, months, and years were fascinating. The doctor taught me all about the human body and how it worked. He would explain to me, from the text, all the data I needed to have a full understanding of what made the body tick. Especially helpful was the information about how muscles grow. The theories I learned provided me with a total and absolute understanding of the nature of muscle, and were the beginnings of what would become the Intensity/Insanity, or Atomic Fitness, principles.

As fate would have it, yet another doorway in my journey to become Mr. America opened when my Uncle John, married to my father's sister, came to visit from Arizona. I had never met anyone like him before. To look at him, it was immediately apparent that he was a man of great distinction. He spoke with authority, while projecting a gentleness and immense understanding in his communication. Uncle John worked at Area 51. I didn't know much about it back then, but I lay on the carpet next to the dinner table listening to Uncle John talk to my parents and was fascinated by his discussion of UFOs and space aliens.

During the week Uncle John stayed with us, I was careful not to miss a single word he said. Even though I was intrigued by the stories of Area 51, I was even more interested in his discussions about time, space, energy, and matter, which, I later learned, were the basics of physics. I don't know why, but somehow I understood there was a connection between what he was saying and my quest to become Mr. America.

Uncle John spoke about experiments involving force, and how the application of force could change time and space, and eventually bring about a measurable change in matter. Matter, I thought, muscle is matter, isn't it? If so, then couldn't the principles of physics, of time, space, and energy, be used to create muscle matter? I couldn't wait for the next opportunity to discuss this insight of mine with Uncle John, and I woke him early the next morning to learn more about these incredible theories, which would become the origins of my Atomic Fitness theory.

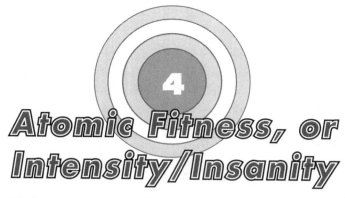

Atomic Fitness, or Intensity/Insanity

The Principles of Time, Space, and Muscle

Well Stevie, I'm pleased to see you're interested in basic physics," Uncle John said encouragingly. I was excited that Uncle John took an interest in me, but I had to be cautious, for looming a few feet away was the ominous figure of my father staring at me with great disapproval. As those long-ago days passed (hard to believe it's now forty years since I first learned the basic principles of mass and force, and how they interact), I continued my talks with Uncle John. They proved incredibly valuable in my quest to learn everything I could about bodybuilding, providing me with knowledge not only of how to build a body but how to do it faster than anyone ever thought possible.

These principles of time, space, and muscle basically changed my life. I applied this system to building my body *and* my mind. This was fortunate, for it was mental fortitude that enabled me to overcome barriers and achieve my titles. More importantly, later in my life, this willpower and mental strength saved my life. . . .

I awakened in a cold and dimly lit hospital room that day. "Where am I? What is this place?" I demanded.

"Calm down, Mr. Michalik. You're in the emergency room at Brunswick Hospital. There was an accident and they brought you here," the attendant explained.

"I need to get going," I insisted. "I'm on my way to L.A. to compete in the contest of my life." I had just won the heavyweight division of the Mr. Universe contest in London, and I had every intention of defending my title in California in the Mr. Olympia contest. I hadn't yet realized that the biggest challenge of my life lay in front of me, and it had nothing to do with bodybuilding.

I tried to stand on my feet. I would have fallen to the ground if it hadn't been for the attendant, who answered my insistence that I had to leave by saying, "You're not going anywhere." Then a cold sweat broke out all over my body as I realized I couldn't feel my legs. They were there, but they were numb. Panic set in, that feeling of total helplessness when you're in a situation you can't do anything about.

"I'm Doctor Illman, an orthopedic surgeon here at Brunswick, and I'll be your doctor," said a man with a soft, determined voice who was standing by my bed.

"I don't need a doctor," I cried out, "I have to go."

As the gravity of my situation began to set in, however, I realized how useless it was to protest. I'm not going anywhere, I thought, I'm really not going anywhere.

It turned out that the accident caused an injury to my back and spine that left me crippled, and not just physically. Something else was crushed— I was suddenly vulnerable. I wasn't immortal after all, at least that's what everyone was trying to tell me. Every conceivable emotion and thought bounced through my head, like Bingo numbers waiting their turn to be counted. When every emotion had its turn to slap me around, I realized no one, not God nor man, was going to help me. Refusing to be less than I am, I decided I would have to conquer this alone, and this was the turning point. My battle had begun, and I would win, or I would die trying. I would never give in.

The rest is history. I defeated the enemy of doubt and frustration. I disagreed with the voices telling me, "You can never . . . " I had used the data of the mind I learned as a child to become Mr. America and Mr. Universe, and I would use it to win this battle as well, and return to the stage. And so I did.

The principles I used to win my titles and return from the dead are the principles of Atomic Fitness. Throughout my career as a professional bodybuilder, I have repeatedly used this method to produce champions in both mind and body. Whether you're a beginner, or have been training for years, these principles can benefit you in your quest for the ultimate physique. But in order to effectively apply the Atomic Fitness method, it is necessary to understand the concepts of the mind, as well as mass and force, which refers to the amount of matter and its ability to resist motion when acted on by a force. Simply put in terms of building muscle, the amount of force applied to muscle equals the amount of mass produced. The less force you apply, the lesser the muscle. The greater the force you apply, the larger and stronger the muscle. Muscle mass has magnitude, or size, which is determined by the muscles' *inability* to handle force. Yes, inability. A muscle that has a lot of power, and can handle force, will *not* be stimulated to grow because the force that muscle experiences is minimal. In order to fully understand this, you must know the basics of physics and how it applies to you and your desire to build muscle. The following definitions are important to learn and understand.

- **ENERGY:** The capacity to do work.
- **FORCE:** The amount of energy or strength applied to an object.
- **MASS:** The measure of a body's resistance to force.
- **WORK:** The transfer of energy when force is applied to an object (a body).
- **TIME:** The ratio of speed over space.
- **SPACE:** The distance between one point and another.

The Atomic Fitness System of training involves all these principles. When applied to exercise, they form the equation below, the secret to building muscle fast.

INTENSITY (the increased amount of work or physical effort)

+ INSANITY (the decreased time, or increased speed, combined with
_____ increased force to cause rapid growth by artificial means)

MASS (the measure of a body's resistance to acceleration)

Force has a quantity, or amount. It can have any magnitude, from a flick to an explosion. In every repetition of your exercise, it is necessary to create as much force as possible. The standard method of exercising with weights requires lifting a heavy weight for a given number of repetitions. This has some validity, but it is limited by the amount of weight a person can lift, which makes progress subservient to the level of strength.

There lies its downfall, and the first limiting factor to building muscle—*strength.* To conquer this, it is necessary to overcome, or bypass, strength and go straight into force. The Atomic Fitness System does just that. The dependence on the strength factor is why the old basic method of weight training takes so long to get results. Strength is largely determined by the body's structure, the inherited soft-tissue connections in the joints, and leverage factors determined by the length of bone in relation to muscle. I have only seen about 2 percent of the training population who have such genetic advantages. The rest were doomed to failure (until now).

To understand why force is more important than strength, you must first understand the structure of muscle and how it responds to force. A muscle is made of fibers, such as those used to make a sweater. Pull out one fiber and little happens. Pull out a whole bunch and the whole sweater falls apart. Muscle fibers work on a similar principle. The number of muscle fibers involved in any given motion is determined by the initial force applied to it. Apply a simple force and only a few muscle fibers respond. The greater the force applied to muscle, the more fibers needed to join in the work.

The optimal scenario is, of course, to recruit all muscle fibers in any given exercise. Before you learn how this is accomplished, however, you need to know the *who, what, why, and how* of it, so you can fully understand the principles, and how the mind plays into combining energy and matter. Understanding all this is crucial to your success, and once you understand, you will build muscle, burn fat, and generally tone up beyond your wildest imagination.

The second limiting factor in building muscle is *endurance*, the ability to withstand stress over time. Again, there is a quagmire. In order to build muscle, you need to put in a lot of time, and time requires endurance. On the other hand, if you put too much time into your training, your endurance will fail and you will not be able to perform at your maximum level. It is also a fact that muscle cannot sustain a long period of work and still grow. There are chemical processes at play that will either enable muscle growth or inhibit it. The Atomic Fitness System has overcome these endurance factors with the principle of maximum effort.

The third limiting factor in building a body, which I cannot emphasize enough, is without a doubt the most important—the *mind factor*. This controls all you need to build your body, whether you are aiming to achieve muscle tone, build muscle, or burn fat. A person's will is what drives success or failure, the ability to bypass pain, and the voices in the head that say it's time to quit. Athletes who fail in their sport do not fail from lack of talent or ability. The failure is in the mind, which transfers that failure to the body. What's known in the sports world as a mind slump is not physiological; its power lies in the mind. Every day, people suffer from this condition, whether it's at work, in the home, or under stress-related conditions such as exercise. Mind slumps seem an unavoidable fact of life—that is, until now. The Atomic Fitness System of mind silencing can, and will, overcome any psychological barriers to your success, especially those obstacles that manifest themselves as pain and an unwillingness to continue.

Psychological pain that manifests as muscle pain prevents fast, lasting results from exercising. Overcoming these sensations is the key to the Atomic Fitness System of training. Once people understand the psychology behind these sensations, they can start to overcome them easily. For example, when you stub your toe, you experience pain. However, the pain is not in your toe, it is actually a psychological manifestation in your brain. It is the same with your muscle. When you learn to control what I call the "fire wall"—the psychological pain sensation you *think* you feel in your muscle—then anything is possible.

Psychological and physiological pain barriers experienced during exercise are known as *phantom sensations,* similar to the phantom-limb phenomena experienced by people with amputations. Such individuals often feel cramps, pain, and tingling sensations in the area of removed appendages, but what they're actually experiencing is the *memory* of sensations. These memories of pain and stress are recorded in the unconscious mind as mental-image pictures.

This also applies to building muscle. The pain experienced while train-

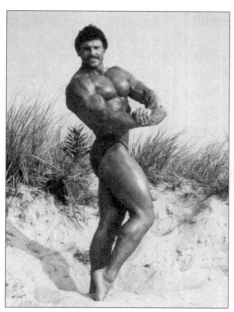 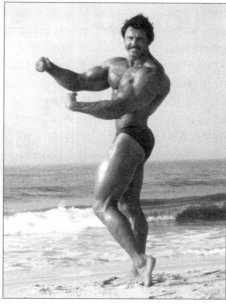

Goal • Barrier of Pain • Success

ing does not originate in the muscle, but rather in the mind, and mental-image pictures of pain and force are stored in the mind as memories. Storing these memories is a survival mechanism the body uses to prepare itself for the next stressful condition, in this case exercise. In order to build your body, it is necessary to overcome these mental images because too many memories of pain can interfere with the ability to build muscle by convincing you to quit. However, if you *increase* the mental images of force and *decrease* those of pain, you can overcome these mental barriers—the optimum scenario would be to create a disproportionate ratio of mental-image pictures in favor of force.

Low-intensity training does just the opposite of this. It creates a ratio of pain to force in favor of pain where the pain memories will become so numerous, they will inhibit your ability to train as hard as you can, ultimately convincing you to quit. On the other hand, a high level of intensity during training allows the muscle to store ten times as many mental-image pictures of force as standard training procedures. (The example of hair waxing can illustrate this concept; if the wax is removed slowly, the pain registered is far greater than if it's removed in one swift motion.)

Due to its rapidity, the Atomic Fitness System delivers a substantially greater level of force than all other alternate training methods. This system creates a high level of stress in the area, convincing the muscle to store as many of these experiences as possible while, at the same time, providing you with the tolerance to overcome these sensations. To achieve this, it is important to fully understand that the sensations experienced are not actually in the muscle, but rather in the mind-brain connection. They are truly originating in the fire wall in your head, and all rapid and permanent gains are achieved beyond this wall. By providing the preferred ratio of force to pain, the Atomic Fitness System provides you with greater potential to overcome this mental barrier. Through years of observation, I've discovered that *anyone*—from construction workers to homemakers, and everyone in between—can break through this wall. It's just a battle between you and your body and a desire to do so.

5

Darwin and the Atomic Fitness System

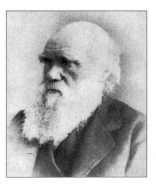

Evolution:
Charles Darwin

D arwin and I make strange companions. We are, after all, 200 years apart. However, I feel Darwin and the Atomic Fitness System of building muscle have remarkable similarities. So, in order to understand the nature of muscle and why it changes, it is important to have a basic understanding of Darwin and his theories.

First, it should be noted that many exercise routines claim to be effective in building muscle, strength, and athletic fitness. Most of these are, in fact, worthless because the trainers switch from routine to routine to find one that works. The only routine that passes the test of time is one that can demonstrate results. A good example of popular but worthless training is the one-body-part-a-day routine—the chest one day, shoulders the next, and so forth, until all the body parts are done. The problem with this method is, by the time you get back to the body part you started with, that muscle has already atrophied back to its original state because it has not received adequate blood circulation, nerve firing, and non-survival stimulation to

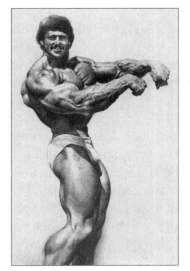

Revolution:
Steve Michalik

change. The key to why this routine fails is its inability to create and maintain a non-survival environment in the muscle, which as we have discussed is necessary to change the muscle. From years of observation, I have learned that after seventy-two-hour periods of no exercise, muscles revert back to their original state (they shrink). I believe there is a monitoring gene that regulates muscle growth through stimulation. If no new non-survival stimulation is delivered to the muscle, the system will withhold the materials necessary to maintain the muscle at that level, for the body does not sense a need.

This brings us to Charles Darwin and his theory of natural selection. Darwin was a nineteenth-century biologist from England who set off to investigate different species and the science, laws, or principles of classifying living organisms in specially named categories based on shapes, characteristics, and natural relationships. This would certainly include muscle, which can be defined as a complex organism because it consists of more than one cell. Muscle cells are biological tissues that perform specific functions, including movement, feeding, growth, reproduction, respiration, and sensitivity to stimuli.

All living beings, including humans, are organisms made up of many other complex organisms. What is of specific interest to this book is the complex organism of muscle tissue. Even though muscle tissue is a symbiotic (living together in close association) part of the body, it is, nevertheless, a separate organism.

Darwin's theory of natural selection can be applied to building muscle as well. Natural selection is considered a large contributing factor in the diversity of species and their genes, and the principles offered by Darwin provide sound explanations of why muscle tissue responds so well to the Atomic Fitness System. Let's look at the principles of Darwin's work, and his theories, as I have applied them.

First, Darwin put forward that all species (all muscle, for our purposes) aim primarily to reproduce and survive, so that they can pass on their genetic information to subsequent generations. When species do this, they tend to produce more offspring, in this case, more muscle tissue. The Atomic Fitness System introduces massive amounts of intense genetic survival information from one generation of muscle cells to the next. When the cell does this, it tends to produce more of itself (offspring), in this case a thicker muscle fiber.

Second, Darwin showed that a lack of resources to nourish individuals leads to competition, decreased population size of species, and failure of some organisms to survive. With living beings, muscle takes precedence over fat. Fat does not survive, muscle does. Training for too long a period of time, or with long rest periods between sets, can cause a lack of available resources to nourish the muscle because there are only so many nutrients in the body. The vital organs, especially the brain and heart, are the first to benefit, and they will compete for the recovery nutrients the muscle needs in order to grow, so muscles starve.

Third, Darwin discovered that the organisms more likely to survive were the ones better suited to their environment. A muscle that survives a workout does not have to change. It is in no danger. Only when a non-survival condition is introduced to the muscle tissue will it change to adapt to this new environment. Continuous non-survival data put upon the muscle will ensure its continuous strength and growth.

The phrase *survival of the fittest* comes from Darwin's observation that organisms most suited to their environment are more likely to survive if the species falls on hard times. A body part that will not grow, or respond to exercise can be said to have "survived the fittest." It has easily adapted to the exercise environment, so it doesn't have to change. The Atomic Fitness System blasts through this consideration and shocks the muscle into new growth.

Finally, according to Darwin, organisms better suited to their environment exhibit desirable characteristics (because their genome is more suitable). Basically, most trainees find it difficult to develop the calves. This is

The Four Basic Types of Tissue in the Body

- **Muscle tissue.** Muscle cells contain filaments that move past one another and change the size of the cell, which is why muscles fall into the category of living organisms. The tissues listed below all influence muscles and fat burning.

- **Epithelial tissue (epithelium).** This tissue absorbs, covers, lines, protects, and secretes.

- **Connective tissue.** This tissue holds everything together. Blood is considered a connective tissue.

- **Nervous tissue.** The cells of this tissue form the brain, spinal cord, and peripheral nervous system.

because that muscle organism is better suited to handle the workload than most other muscle areas. The calf muscle has desirable characteristics suited for survival because it is the first muscle you used to a large degree when you started to walk (just observe a baby).

Over the years, this calf muscle strengthened itself and adapted to stress. Today, just by walking around, every step that puts weight on the calf reinforces this. Only new, intensive, environmental stimulation through the Atomic Fitness System of training will make the calves grow. There are other muscle groups that are also difficult to develop due to heredity factors built into the body from past stress in those areas. This is generational-ancestral adaptation syndrome (GAAS), where past generations have used certain muscle groups over an extended period of time and have learned to adapt to the environment. Normally, any system that has adapted will not change (this applies to fat-burning as well), but the Atomic Fitness System can force new genetic considerations and overcome GAAS.

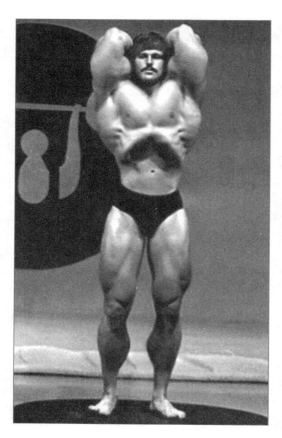

Survival of the fittest—
He who survives . . .
wins.

This Darwinian concept of survival adaptation is useful in understanding how to build muscle—those that adapt and change survive, while those that do not adapt and change stay the same and succumb. In nature, the bear is an example of this. In the distant past, when the earth turned very cold, bears that grew heavy fur and thick layers of fat survived. Those that stayed the same perished, as did some early humans. Due to changes in weather and dangers from the environment, humans living in caves could not hunt consistently. Their bodies had to adapt to store food for long periods of time. Those whose systems adapted by storing food as fat survived; the rest became extinct. This same principle applies to building muscle and to fat metabolism. Any external, non-survival stimulation to the muscle must cause it to change so it can adapt and survive. This is absolutely proven by those who possess large muscles and demonstrate great strength and ability.

It is also important to note that the greater the stimulus (of a non-survival nature), the greater the change. Those muscles that do not change have adapted *too* well and will resist anything you throw at them—until now, that is. The Atomic Fitness System can cause any area to react to change.

The same holds true for fat burning with aerobic exercise. If you do the same aerobic activity too often, your body will adapt to it and slow your metabolism down to a crawl in an effort to survive. The minute you become aerobically efficient, you will start to get fat again. Perfect examples of this are aerobics and spin classes. Yes, they will improve you cardio fitness and you will become efficient at them. However, when this happens, your body is no longer in a non-survival mode, so it doesn't need to change or burn fat anymore. Since the body learns to anticipate consistent levels of threat, it will adopt a survival posture from past experiences and will no longer perceive the activity as a threat. The only way to keep your body changing is to create different non-survival techniques. This is what Atomic Fitness is all about. This is why you plateau, why you fail, why you get discouraged, and why you ultimately quit. I will not let this happen.

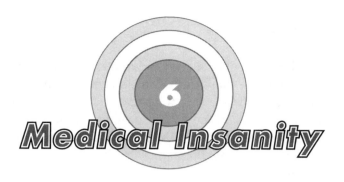

Medical Insanity

Almost everything you have learned about health, nutrition, and exercise is erroneous. A bold statement, but think about this: the doctors who are supposed to provide the pinnacle of good health also personally battle heart disease, weight gain, and every other ailment they say they can cure. How can this be? If doctors and fitness experts can't even save their own lives, how can they save yours? Oh yes, they do their best in their specialties, but to fully help anyone who's ill, one must understand how the different methodologies fit together, and when it comes to this, most M.D.s are simply lost. Truthfully, the only person who can help you is *you*.

The fact is, the human body wants to heal itself, and although there are a few enlightened physicians who are willing to seek and administer genuine therapy to help the body along in this regard, the larger part of the medical profession hasn't a clue regarding muscle building or weight loss, and they know even less about nutrition. Most doctors are driven by drug-oriented beliefs, which blind them to more natural methods. But with specific nutritional intake provided by you through proper eating and exercise, your body has the ability to make the necessary adjustments to overcome most any condition. The body is basically a mobile machine. It's designed to move and be driven. This is where proper exercise comes in. This concept is neglected by most "experts," particularly those with M.D. after their names.

Unfortunately, too much of our nation is still in the Dark Ages when it comes to understanding what our bodies require to achieve maximum fitness and health. The myths, lies, and false data that permeate this area are astounding. The millions of programs, routines, and scientific data available to help us build muscle are basically useless. I recently had a heated discussion about the beneficial effects of high-intensity training with one of those experts. This doctor was convinced that established scientific evidence disproved my theory. He, of course, had to be right with scientific evidence on his side. At this point, I reminded him that before it was challenged by Galileo, the scientifically accepted theory was that the sun and all the planets revolved around the earth. Also, Einstein's theory of relativity, though good at the time, has currently been expanded upon and challenged by quantum physics. This is not to mention all the other great minds who agreed to disagree. The point is, I urge you to take the time to assimilate the powerful information contained in this book so you can assure yourself the quality of life achieved by good health and the mental ability to achieve your goals.

A body that is allowed to fall from its optimum state will fail on some level. Everyone's body constantly battles the toxins ingested and inhaled from a polluted outside environment. Drugs and most surgeries are not the answers, only a desperate last resort. The truth, as I see it, is that what people eat is killing them. The blood, spinal fluid, and saliva of healthy metabolisms are more alkaline, whereas the fluids of those who are sick are more acidic, with a low pH level and a metabolism that is a disaster in the mak-

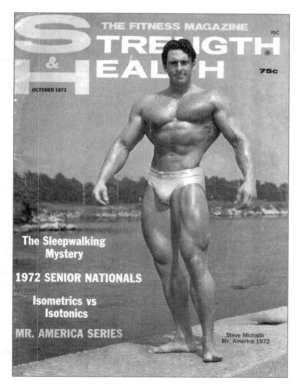

Scientific evidence proves . . . *nothing*. The demonstration of ability is the only proof.

ing: most degenerating metabolisms result in an inability to build muscle, burn fat, fight fatigue, and recover from exercise.

Toxins in the body are responsible for causing most illnesses and inhibiting physical progress. The presence of toxins, and your body's inability to handle them, impedes progress in everything from improving your general health to achieving a championship physique. Toxins are silent killers. They are the barriers to physical and mental survival, and they have been a part of you since the day you were born. As you grew, they grew too, causing childhood illness and disease. As you matured, they continued to multiply, causing further illness and disease. Unless they're eliminated, they will eventually be the cause of your death.

Highly intense, properly executed exercise, along with a sound nutritional program, can go a long way in handling these toxins. It works like this: genetically, each person has stronger and weaker areas in her or his body. As you have lived your life, and built up stress, both mental and physical, your body has accumulated toxins. They have congregated in the weakest areas of your body because that is where they get the least resistance. Fat is a favorite site for toxins, as is unused muscle. When enough toxins have accumulated in a part of your body, they manifest themselves in the form of a disease that is indigenous to that part of your body, and they prevent muscle growth and healthy cellular growth and repair. According to a few of the more enlightened doctors, there are no incurable diseases. What can't be cured are incurable viewpoints.

You owe it to yourself to keep an open mind about all new data and constantly look for truly effective therapies. If you are well informed, you can then agree to disagree with currently well-established scientific facts and learn more timeless facts.

My system provides powerful, priceless information. Its effectiveness has been demonstrated by myself and others, and continues to prove its validity with my clients who range from homemakers to professional businesspeople to champion bodybuilders. I urge you to give my system your best attention and also seek out others who have spent their lives searching out the truth. It is a fact that people are influenced by others in society. The established viewpoints that certain authority figures constantly pound out are reminders of how lives are being manipulated. Remember, as far as your well-being is concerned, it's up to you to discover the facts and take full responsibility for yourself. From my vantage point, most doctors really *don't* know, and don't want you to know that they don't know, and most personal trainers and personal fitness gurus don't have a clue either.

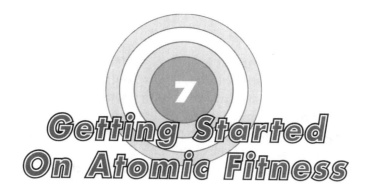

Getting Started On Atomic Fitness

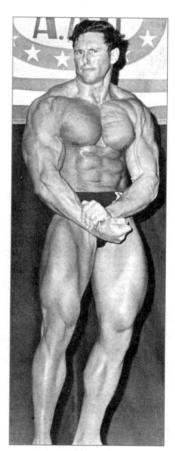

You are what you believe.

If you absorb nothing else from this book, know with certainty that all of your success starts and ends with you, and that you will become what you believe.

Ask yourself these questions:

- Who is most important to you?

- Who do you blame for your failures?

- Who is responsible for your successes?

- Who doesn't live up to their agreements?

- Who is responsible for putting negative viewpoints in your head?

If you search hard enough, and look honestly, you will find that the answer to each question is *you*. If you learn nothing else in this universe, understand this and teach it to your children.

The most important lessons I learned about becoming a champion involved how I felt about me. Nothing you encounter in life means more than how you feel about yourself. Consciously or unconsciously, you are most critical of yourself. This self-criticism is the basis for failure, the lack of positive viewpoints, and uncompleted projects. The pursuit of any goal requires self-trust and abandoning the shame/blame/ regret syndrome. The basis of all reality is that you believe in self and agree with it. Whatever viewpoint you put in front of yourself, you will gravitate to it. You are a creative being, capable of incredible things. And more than any other being on earth, you have the ability to achieve anything you can imagine. What a waste of a gift to drown this ability in lakes of doubt and self-pity.

No matter what you are trying to accomplish, if you keep a positive viewpoint, you will get there. Nothing can stop you except you. Sure, there are barriers in life that try to interfere with your goals and purposes, but barriers are not stops. They're just life's little pauses to get you to look and see what has just happened and formulate a plan of attack to push forward, past the barrier.

Life is a game. Your purposes are part of that game. All games require barriers or else there would be no game. There are no failures, only opportunities to observe the obvious and choose a course of action to conquer and destroy obstacles. Expect nothing to be easy. If it were, the end product would be worthless.

Never let fear get in the way of success. Fear results from a lack of data, from not understanding something. Research that data and you will find the fear disappears.

Knowledge conquers every time. Your brain is like a computer. It reacts to the information it is given, causing biological changes in your body and thinking process. Program in wrong, or false, data and you will react to it. Program it with true and positive data, and your body and mind can only gravitate to positive viewpoints. The voices of doubt in your head are only the echoes of past experiences that don't apply to the here and now. Leave those old viewpoints to the past, and move forward in the present time, creating new, positive ideas and viewpoints.

Let's face it, you're the most important person you know. You count the most. Selfishness and pride are good, positive qualities, and don't let anyone tell you differently. If you are in shape and look and feel good about yourself, you will act differently. You will have energy and vitality and the ability to create anything. There will be nothing that can hold you back.

The price of freedom is your willingness to defeat any and all viewpoints that do not contribute to your success. The reward is the regaining of self. Make every thought in every day count. Seek no counsel for your true

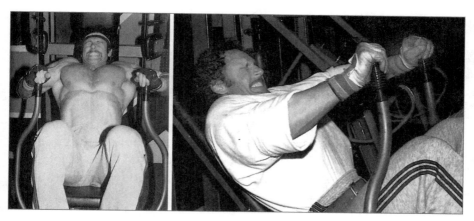

Total mind supremacy. Do anything it takes to win.

beliefs. Believe in self. Plan your moves. Don't let others move you. The time is now. Commit to self. Remember, you are what you believe. Life is consistently pushing back against you, so you must never stop pushing forward. The moment you do, even for a moment, life will crush you.

GENERAL PREPARATORY STAGE

I believe that unless people are generally fit, they will have little success in achieving their goals. Therefore, the initial phase of this, as in any exercise program, is designed primarily to get them in shape and form a foundation for the intense exercise to come.

The goal is to strive for all-around physical fitness. The preconditioning and beginning routines are "primer" workouts devoted to conditioning all major joints, ligaments, muscles, and other support structures, with special attention paid to areas of body weakness. I emphasize a variety of exercises, with volume as a key factor. Dumbbells are the preferred tool to begin with because they allow joints and muscles their full range of motion. At this point, I cannot overstate the importance of building your cardiorespiratory and aerobic fitness, which is best accomplished by slow, gradual progression on aerobic equipment that takes you from fat burning to more of a cardio effect. The optimum goal will be to achieve 80 percent of the maximum levels. Start out slow and build up to them. As you progress, I recommend some strength training of your muscles to prevent injuries. Muscles serve as a buffer for the joints, and if they are weak, damage to the joints will occur. Your target heart rate should be as follows: 220 minus your age multiplied by 80 percent. The result of this equation is your *capacity*. You can check this with a doctor knowledgeable in sports medicine whom you trust.

Depending on your starting level, the preparatory stage should last anywhere from two weeks to three months, after which you gradually make the transition into the next phase. If any general weakness exists in any area, some specialized conditioning for that area should be introduced. If you refer to the anatomy diagrams in Figures 7.1 and 7.2, and coordinate them with the exercises specified for the targeted body part, you can develop a specific strengthening routine.

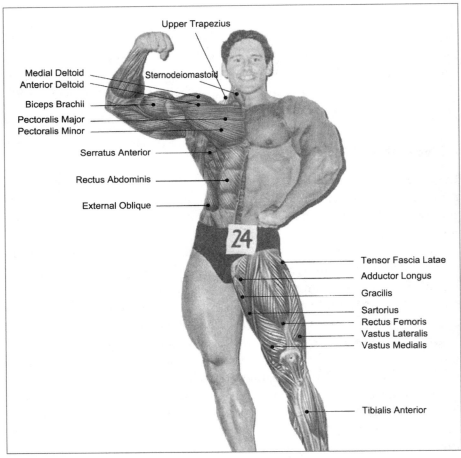

Figure 7.1. Anantomy diagram (anterior)

When your body can handle the preparatory stage easily—that is, with moderate effort, speed, and mental clarity—you can then proceed to the next level. At this point, the volume and the intensity of the exercise should increase. This is a very demanding period in your training because what I am basically requiring is for you to disagree with reality and break into a new level of fitness, musculature, and vitality. This is your opportunity to raise above the old self into a new you. Your speed, strength, and determination will be tested. Remember, the way out of your weakness is to go through it. No backing off. No backing down. Your body will resist, you will persevere. You are reading this book, and it just may be the best thing you have ever done for yourself—now use it.

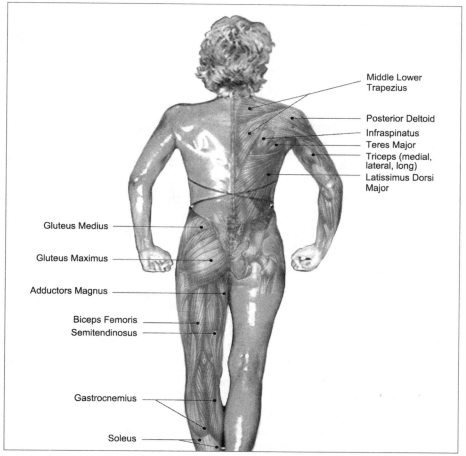

Figure 7.2. Anantomy diagram (posterior)

Flexibility

Flexibility is the term used to describe your range of motion in a joint. It is a measurement of how far you can move your limbs and torso around each joint. In the gyms I have visited, I found an obsession for stretching. Trainers and coaches would mistakenly have their trainees stretch before everything, from brushing their teeth to lovemaking. Before and after, morning, noon, and night, they would have you believe that stretching is an absolute necessity. But is all that stretching really necessary? Russian and European researchers have concluded that your level of flexibility is predetermined by your genes, and you can achieve flexibility only to that biological degree. If a person performs her or his exercises with a full range of motion, using little resistance, that area will naturally reach its own maximum level of flexibility, and no amount of stretching will change that. Your body will stretch only so far and no further. There are structural limitations on everyone, and attempts to increase flexibility beyond your natural ability can be a dangerous scenario for the ligaments. The elasticity of the muscles and tendons protect the joints from injury. If you exceed this limitation by overstretching, causing your ligaments to overstretch, you will lose your buffer against injury. Your ligaments will remain in this state, the joints they hold together will weaken, and injury will follow.

The preconditioning phase of Atomic Fitness is primarily designed to maximize your muscle tone and prevent such an occurrence. If you have to stretch, let me give you a few pointers. First, never do what most trainers would have you do, which is to slowly sustain a stretch where your muscles are at their maximum length and you're experiencing pain. If you feel pain, it's a warning sign that something is wrong. Your body is telling you it has had enough. But, adhering to the no-pain, no-gain theory, some trainers feel the need to take you beyond this point. They're only asking for trouble because most injuries occur at the extreme range of motion. This action should be avoided, both in your flexibility and exercise routines.

In addition to the above concerns, Russian research has concluded that certain forms of stretching may actually *cause* injury, rather than prevent it. For example, take placing your leg up on a bar and reaching for your foot. With this action, the risk of hamstring and spinal injury is real, and long-term use of this action may cause permanent damage.

Unfortunately, people tend to behave like cattle or sheep, going through life passively accepting another's lead. Never be part of the herd. Break away. Walk alone, walk free. You're in the Atomic Zone now.

Body Fitness

Body fitness usually means physical fitness or conditioning. I like to think of it as mind and body endurance. I can't emphasize enough the necessity of cardiovascular fitness. This allows your circulatory system to sustain exercise at a high level of intensity over an extended period of time. And the ability to supply oxygen to muscle cells is a critical factor in the pursuit of a lean, muscular, toned physique. Transporting oxygen to the areas you're

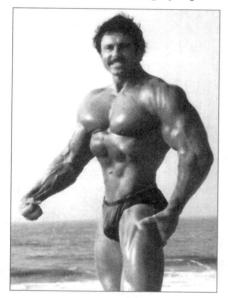

training will be the limiting physical factor in any exercise program.

There are also mental factors at play. The soreness you feel after training sessions doesn't necessarily indicate you've worked hard. What it most definitely does mean is that your heart and lungs could not sustain an adequate ratio of oxygen to energy. Therefore, the energy in your muscle, in this case glycogen or sugar, will not be fully utilized, leaving an acid behind in that area. *This* is the pain or soreness you feel. A well-conditioned body should *never* get sore. Both high-intensity training and aerobics are intended to increase your body's ability to take in oxygen, and more important, to exhale the unused oxygen in the system. Any leftover oxygen, not absorbed or exhaled, will stay in the lungs, causing a shortness of breath. It's your body's desperate attempt to rid itself of the unused oxygen. When you're breathing hard during exercise, you have what is known as an oxygen debt. This is the precursor to muscular failure. In connection with this, if your breathing becomes difficult while you're doing your fat-burning exercises, you're in oxygen debt, which means you're working your muscles and burning sugar, *not* fat. To repeat, you're not burning fat—you're using sugar and losing muscle.

WHAT THE ATOMIC FITNESS SYSTEM WILL DO FOR YOU

The innumerable, inefficient systems of exercise thrust on you, along with all sorts of extraordinary bicycles, springs, walking machines, and similar apparatus, are alleged to lead users directly into vim, vigor, vitality, and a classic physique—*not so*. The ineffectiveness of these systems is proven by how quickly they're given up on, only to be utilized as clothes hangers and dust collectors.

The Atomic Fitness System is a truly effective way to stimulate the action of the muscles, improve blood circulation, and also improve the coordination of nerves and muscles. The chief value of physical activity is to stimulate the general chemistry and physiology of the body through its effect on circulation and elimination of waste. This is why a person feels better after working out with Atomic Fitness routines.

Everyone should have sufficient strength in their muscles to carry out the ordinary activities of life and to permit exceptional use of them in times of emergency. Atomic Fitness does this and more. For young adults, Atomic Fitness has the benefit of stimulating body growth. For mature adults, it is the fountain of youth. Before undertaking any kind of strenuous physical activity, however, let your doctor determine the capacity of your heart.

Why is it important to do Atomic Fitness? Those who do not engage in force training do not experience optimum health and vitality. Atomic Fitness provides what is known as maximum tone, which gives muscle the ability to respond when called on, especially in an emergency.

Atomic Fitness develops tissues so they will be capable of efficiently performing their intended functions forever. This is done by increasing the circulation of the blood, thereby aiding in the nourishment of individual cells in the body. Improved circulation also helps remove waste material from the body. Furthermore, Atomic Fitness also increases the depth and rate of breathing, which gives the red blood cells more oxygen to carry, and helps eliminate carbon dioxide.

The chief benefits of Atomic Fitness are that it increases the ability of the body to do physical work, lessens fatigue, increases endurance, and produces perfection of movement. Increased work increases the need for oxygen, causing an increased rate of deeper breathing. Young-adult trainees need more exercise because their bodies are still growing, so they take in more oxygen and give out more waste matter than the mature adult.

Atomic Fitness improves the quality of the body as well as its performance. It helps coordinate the muscles so they perform more efficiently and require less energy. The warming-up process enables bodybuilders to reach their maximum requirement, and prevents shortness of breath and discomfort, which usually precedes what athletes call the second wind.

Atomic Fitness increases *vital capacity*, which is the amount of air that can be handled by the lungs. The average athlete has a capacity of four to five quarts of air, in contrast to three quarts for a non-athlete. An increase in endurance, resulting from good physical training, is shown by the fact that the onset of fatigue is delayed.

One of the most important aspects of Atomic Fitness is the practice of correct form. The system will not be effective if you don't learn to train correctly, vigorously, and in good form. Perform the exercises with enthusiasm. Count out loud. Go entirely through each set with drive. Investing your time this way cannot help but pay big dividends.

WHERE AND WHEN TO BEGIN

In any exercise program, there are guidelines to follow. The suggestions below have all been devised using a scientific approach, and contain sound advice that should be adhered to when embarking on the exercise programs provided in Chapter 8.

1. Before starting an exercise program, check your general health with a physician.

2. Keep consistent written records of your progress in weight and measurements. Take pictures if possible.

3. Note any previous injuries you may have had.

4. Exercise on a gradient level, a little at a time, building up to high intensity.

5. Stay focused. Always keep your goals and purposes in front of you.

6. In conditioning training, always do a total body workout, working the largest muscles first.

7. Never exercise with heavy weights. It is best to increase the intensity instead.

8. Eliminate bad habits such as drinking alcohol, inadequate sleep, and smoking.

9. Challenge yourself.

10. Exercise in a pleasant atmosphere.

11. Understand the psychology of the mind.

12. Study the philosophy of knowing.

13. Understand the dynamics of the body.

14. Never waver.

Anyone, regardless of age, can benefit from Atomic Fitness, but prepubescent trainees should concentrate on a conditioning program rather than weight training (see the Preconditioning Routine and Beginning Routine I in Chapter 8). They should also be advised not to test their strength with heavy, one-repetition exercises, since there may be some danger of injuring the soft cartilagelike growth centers in the bone.

Beginners should follow the Preconditioning Routine (see Chapter 8). It might be a good idea, however, for beginners to use only about two-thirds the amount of weight they would be able to handle if they were to make a maximum effort.

Basic Bodybuilding Rules

Rule 1. Always remember to warm up sufficiently before training. Work your way up, using a system of graduated levels of weight and speed, progressively getting stronger.

Rule 2. Seek advice from *no one*. Keep your own counsel. There is something to gain from asking questions, but the final decision must be your own. You are an individual and must determine your own capabilities, so it is most important to think for yourself.

Rule 3. Never miss a workout. If you plan three workouts every week, then allow nothing to keep you from your commitment. Continue to have enthusiasm and be patient. A quality product requires this. You can't fail.

Rule 4. Always use the Atomic Fitness System. Your muscles should be coaxed into harder work. You have to shock the body constantly with more force, Atomic style.

Rule 5. Enjoy normal, healthy hygiene. Get plenty of good, wholesome food. Obtain enough sleep so you awake refreshed. Maintain a tranquil mind and enjoy social recreation.

Rule 6. Remember to breathe. The more oxygen you can absorb, the more endurance your muscles will have. Also, deep breathing promotes fat burning and muscle healing.

Confusion in the mind of the beginner is universal, and indeed worthy of more consideration than it has received. What most beginners are seeking is simplified terminology and a concrete program of physical development. But before I attempt to offer any plan to clear up some of this confusion, I want to assure everyone that there is indeed a miracle system, which basically consists of hard work, dedication, perseverance, patience, and a complete understanding of the body and mind. Any individuals just starting Atomic Fitness must always use moderation and should concern themselves with conditioning the body in order to support more weight as their skills progress. The same principle applies in all Atomic Fitness exercises, regardless of how they are performed.

How to Breathe

The average person breathes from seventeen to twenty times per minute. Women breathe a bit more rapidly than men. All of us breathe more rapidly when standing than sitting. The amount of air taken in with a single breath averages three quarts for grown men, and two quarts for grown women. With that said, in most exercises, it really doesn't matter too much how you breathe, as long as you breathe rhythmically with each repetition, and avoid holding your breath. You should try to exhale during the phase of an exercise in which muscular contraction or exertion seems to interfere with inhalation. In sit-ups, for example, you should exhale while rising to a sitting position. Holding your breath and straining while your abdominal muscles are contracted could result in a hernia or even a blackout. Remember, oxygen is the key to a hard workout.

Resting After a Workout

When you have completed your workout, try to cool down for a half hour or so. Your heart pumps a greater volume of blood when the body is moving instead of just sitting around. Champion bodybuilders speed their recovery by tapering off their workouts with light exercise, so that muscular contractions will pump fresh blood though the fatigued muscles. However, until you become more accustomed to your training, don't force yourself too vigorously. It's important to remember that you only recover when you rest.

If you train regularly, you'll find that Atomic Fitness will actually relieve the fatigue of a sedentary lifestyle, and you'll have a lot more energy for everyday living.

THE FUNCTIONS OF MUSCLES—SOME FACTS AND MYTHS

There are many misconceptions being promoted about prime muscles and their functions, so it is important to clear up any myths and misinformation in order to apply effective training principles in your routine. Muscles increase their usable strength as they change their positions from full extension to full contraction. In order to achieve this goal, though, you must clearly understand the muscles' function.

Muscles have numerous functions, but we are only concerned here with the primary and secondary functions of the major muscle groups. For example, one myth is that the bicep muscle is used for bending the arm up or curling a weight. This is, in fact, the secondary function of the bicep. Its primary function is to twist the hand, or, as referred to in physiological circles, activate the supination of the wrist. In the case of the right hand, the bicep action is right to left, and with the left hand, it is left to right. It has been proven that a muscle, the bicep in this case, is strongest and will develop fastest by isometrically twisting—that is, rotating the hand against an immovable object—at the end of each contraction. Each exercise has its own value, but performing the wrong motion will limit the ability to use all the muscle fibers. In the case of the bicep, twisting your hand, as explained above, will develop this area to its fullest.

Another widely promoted myth is that muscles have the ability to perform both pushing and pulling motions. This is a fallacy. Although there appear to be situations that contradict this rule, muscles perform work *only* by pulling, not pushing. One muscle group that falls into this category is the pectoral or chest muscles. The pectoral muscles are located directly below the scapula bone, just above the rib cage. The function of these muscles appears to be to *push* the arms up, away from the chest position (as in a bench-press exercise). How is it possible for the pectoral muscles to perform work in two apparently opposite directions? The answer is, of course, that they cannot, though they appear to do so. What actually occurs is, by contracting the pectoral muscles, you raise the elbows to a position where other muscles can straighten the arm, giving the appearance of a push when the muscles have really been performing a pulling function.

An example known to most bodybuilders is the misconception of how the *latissimus dorsi* muscles work (these are the muscles located right under the armpit, going along the side of the body). These muscles are believed to grow wider and thicker during exercises with a wide grip, under the sincere but mistaken idea that such a grip will provide more stretch and more width for this muscle area. Actually, if you study the range of movement and the position of hands to muscle, you'll find that a narrower grip will provide more stretch, and work the muscle under a greater range of movement, providing a full extension. As I said, muscles increase their usable strength as they change their position from one of full extension to one of full contraction. Therefore, a narrow grip is far more effective than a wider grip for a wider muscle.

I believe one of the greatest misconceptions in bodybuilding and exercise is the purpose of what is commonly known as the squat. It is believed that the primary function of the squat is building the upper leg. This is simply not true. It is, however, by far one of the best butt exercises. The reason for this is that if you study the function of the thigh and buttocks muscles, it is apparent that, with the squat, the thighs cannot perform most of the work. Rather, the stress is on the lower back and the buttocks muscles of the body.

To explain further, it's apparent that a muscle grows bigger and stronger when direct resistance is placed upon it. When performing a squat, the weight is held across the shoulders and the pressure is directed straight down. The resistance, therefore, is placed on the hip joints surrounded by the buttocks' muscles. In order for the resistance to be placed on the thigh muscle, you would have to lean back, keeping the hips and back in a straight line while coming all the way up, and all the way down. If you ever tried this movement, you know it's physically impossible without falling backward. You can try to compensate for this by holding the weight in front, in what is referred to as a front squat. Still, the buttocks muscles must work 80 percent of the time to move the torso in line with the thighs, and the thigh frontal muscle must also, at the same time, move the lower legs forward. This exertion accounts for 20 percent of the effort in the squat. It is, therefore, my contention that you are trying to get the most out of your exercise with the least amount of exertion and effort. The squat does not conform to this standard. In effect, the frontal thigh muscles require what is commonly known as a thigh extension machine for the best direct exercise of that area, and the buttocks muscles are best served by doing the squat.

Since these examples indicate that key major muscular structures do not perform the functions most people think they do, I recommend for a clear understanding that you study the function of every muscle. What I try to stress is that it is important for each individual to try and do exercises in a position that offers the greatest resistance in the contraction, while still providing maximum resistance throughout the entire movement. Those who are interested in reaching maximum development can do so quite easily.

Conventional barbells or dumbbells can be used to the fullest if you study the muscles, learn their functions, and apply the proper exercise position for their use. Information is your ally and misinformation is your enemy—go Atomic.

WHY RESISTANCE TRAINING IS A MUST

How does weight training build your muscles? What is the actual physical process that takes place when weight training is employed to build the body? To fully understand how resistance training works, it's necessary to understand the physical structure of muscle tissue and how this structure is altered by weight training.

Muscles are made up of fibers. These fiber tissues are strands woven together to create a whole mass. What may appear to be a single bulging muscle is, in fact, a great number of tissue fibers. In terms of size, the thicker muscles of the body, such as the thighs and back, have much larger quantities of these fibers than the smaller muscles of the arms and shoulders—and not only are these fibers thicker and heavier, they are also far more numerous.

When you use weights to build up and strengthen your muscles, good things happen. The terms *pumped up* or *pumping muscle* refer to the swelling surrounding the muscle being worked, and this is due to rapidly increasing blood flow into that area. The body always sends a fresh supply of blood to any area of exertion to supply the working area with the nutrients and oxygen needed to carry out its function, while also carrying away broken-down cells from that area so the nutrients can build up and help the area become stronger, more useful, and more shapely.

Your body has been designed to meet the demands placed on it. When any level of resistance is placed on a muscle, the body sets up an existing level of muscle development. This existing level of development can be changed by using the Atomic Fitness methods of training that cause the muscles to overload and tear down in response to the demand placed on them. As this happens, the body will receive a signal to rush nutrients and oxygen from the bloodstream to this particular area of stress. The muscle then swells with nutrients. Since your body knows its business, it sends more than is needed to rebuild this broken-down tissue. This condition should occur after several repetitions of any given exercise, and it is what is referred to as pumped up. A note to remember is that the breaking down of tissue will occur only when you *overwork* your existing level of development. If you don't, then you're only doing what your body is already capable of, and no message will be sent to relieve it with nutrients and rebuilding materials.

You must have maximum intensity to stimulate maximum growth. Maximum intensity does not refer to using excessive amounts of weight, but rather to exerting the greatest amount of effort with force and speed in the shortest amount of time. It is not necessary to train in a dangerous fashion, using heavy weights, to attain maximum-possible intensity.

Muscular injuries result when the pulling force exerted exceeds the breaking strength of some part of the muscular structure. For example, if you are capable of producing one hundred pounds of force in a pressing movement, and if the breaking strength of your shoulder or deltoid muscle attachments is close to seventy-five pounds or less, then you are sure to injure yourself if you perform this maximum-possible press.

A unique function of the muscle is that it can hold greater force once it has been contracted than during the contraction itself. Using the barbell curl as an example, you can resist much more force on the downward motion than you can possibly hope to curl on the way up. On the downward motion, you can literally stop the weight and delay the force, holding your position against a tremendous resistance and producing an incredible effect.

There are three different levels of strength—an upward strength, a holding strength, and a downward strength—and each has a level of intensity all its own. In order for a muscle to achieve its maximum strength and development, you must try to work the greatest intensity on all three levels. It's important to remember that the intensity of an exercise is determined by the amount of effort exerted at a particular time during a movement, not by the amount of weight being used. A simple example of this would be to curl the same weight at different speeds. If you performed this exercise with seventy-five pounds in ten seconds, the intensity would be low. On the other hand, if you curled that same seventy-five pounds in three seconds, then the intensity would certainly be very high.

I hope I am convincing you that the actual amount of exercise is meaningless unless the intensity of the work is very high. An example I use to further explain this concept compares the muscles of long-distance runners to those of sprinters. A long-distance runner can run for hours and hours, over hills and valleys, putting out a tremendous amount of work, and if his muscles were examined, they would consist of long, thin tissue fibers. On the other hand, a sprinter, who runs as hard as he can for a short distance, working as hard as he can in the shortest period of time, would have muscles that are large and thickly developed.

Intensity of effort is good—anything that increases the intensity of an exercise will greatly improve it. Excessive amount of exercise is bad—any excessive amount of exercise exhausts your recovery ability and makes growth impossible. Too much exercise may even result in a loss of the size, strength, and beauty of the muscle.

Just as it should be understood that simply because you can stand a large amount of exercise doesn't mean it will produce much in the way of worthwhile results, it should also be understood that you cannot *stand much exercise if the intensity is high. That is unless you've conquered the "must-fail" mechanism of the mind and agree to a new reality.*

EXERCISE CONSIDERATIONS

In any sport, if you want to increase your skill, your strength, or your inherited ability, you need to challenge yourself to go beyond your current level of achievement, or what is already easy for you. And the rules are the same for stimulating muscle growth. You must constantly attempt what seems impossible. Since low-intensity exercise produces no stimulation and few results, if you want maximum possible growth, an effort approaching momentary existing levels of muscle failure is absolutely required. Many bodybuilders and others seeking to be champions justify their easy workouts on the grounds that they do more. They compensate by doing more sets, more exercises, and training more days a week, with longer hours, which, we have shown, is actually contrary to the laws of development.

Simply adding more exercise to your current routine will never produce the results that are possible from exercising harder. Regardless of the additional exercise, most trainees quickly fall into a rut where their workouts almost totally deplete their recovery ability. It takes them years to produce results that could have been produced in months. Once you have a clear understanding of how the body works, it will be obvious that the Atomic Fitness System is the best one for you.

My aim is to teach you the proper way of training and dispel the belief that more is better. Hard work is best. Everyone would gain from decreasing the time they spend exercising. The Atomic Fitness System is uniquely designed to compress time and space, while large amounts of energy create change in the muscle. You'll find your greatest results in the compression of time instead of in long, drawn-out daily workouts.

Brief, intensive training is an absolute requirement for producing the best possible results from exercise. Yet, almost all currently active trainees devote at least five times as much weekly training time to their workouts as necessary, while producing little or nothing in the way of results. For every hundred trainees, there's probably only one who is presently training correctly. Most trainees seem mainly concerned with daily training time and are willing to devote any amount of time to their workouts, in the belief that such marathon workouts will speed their progress. The opposite is true—long, frequent workouts substantially retard progress. A reduction in training time on the part of all trainees would result in an immediate improvement in their rate of progress.

The best results are produced when the exercises are as hard and fast as

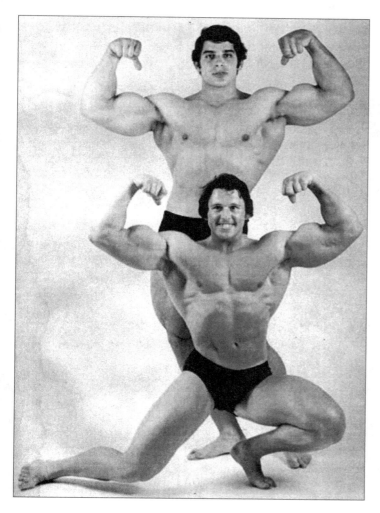

You are responsible for all you've become.

Mr. Universe, Lou Ferrigno; Mr. America, Steve Michalik

Advice for Successful Training

To produce the best possible results, a trainee should follow this advice.

1. It should be your goal to always look for signs of progress and always attempt to produce this progress, with "progress" being the key word. Use cheating movements, or what are commonly called cheating principles, only after you are no longer able to perform your strict reps. Otherwise, you'll only be cheating yourself and the muscle.

2. Pay attention to form and style. Don't degenerate into just going through the movements. You will lower the intensity and also your results. Follow the instructions as described in the routines section in Chapter 8.

3. Never select the easiest exercises. Always perform the hardest exercises in the hardest manner possible. If an exercise is performed in a style that makes it easier, it's almost always less productive.

4. Even if you have completed your selected guideline number of repetitions, your set is never properly done until no further movement of the resistance is possible. If you are doing presses, you are done only when you can no longer move the bar from your shoulders. A set of curls is only complete when the weight will not come up from your thighs no matter how hard you try.

5. If you perform more repetitions than you have selected, then the intensity is too easy. You need to adjust the resistance.

6. Judge your progress, not only by the tape and the scale, but by looking at yourself. Unless you are measuring every inch of every body part, it is impossible to measure growth or reduction on a tape or scale.

7. In general, a clear understanding of progress should come from your performance of the routine. It's certain that your muscles

will be at least twice as fit as they were at the start of any exercise program when you can perform twice as many repetitions with twice as much resistance in half the time.

8. You should never get discouraged by comparing yourself with others. It is impossible to make such comparisons on a rational basis because too many factors—such as bone structure, heredity, muscle insertions, and other variables—are involved. Your body is personal. Love it, respect it, and appreciate your progress.

9. When you sleep, your body systems work as a team and should be treated that way. You don't think of your arms sleeping one hour, your legs sleeping the next, and then maybe your kidneys taking a rest for an hour or two. That would seem ridiculous. Only a deep sleep can bring about the physical change you desire.

10. Spot reduction of fatty tissue is a fairy tale, a physical impossibility. Build the muscles of your abdominal area by training them exactly the same way you exercise your other muscles. There is *absolutely nothing* in the way of artificial aids that will help the situation. All that really matters is your overall consumption of calories—energy output, food input. This will result in fat loss. (*See* Chapters 13–17.)

11. Do not make the mistake of trying to add muscular size by bulking up—adding fatty tissue. This fatty tissue is not muscle and cannot become muscle. Fat cells can be increased in number, and once added, new fat cells can only be completely removed by surgery. You can reduce the size of fat cells, but you cannot entirely remove them.

12. Your training time includes only the time actually devoted to working against resistance—the total training time minus resting time. Your training pace is determined by the delay between sets and the speed of movement. Speed and the collapsing of space are absolutely necessary in building muscle.

possible. In practice, the most productive method of training requires the utilization of one or more training routines. A resistance should be selected that will permit the performance of a given number of repetitions. Each set should be carried out to failure, to the point where even the slightest degree of additional movement is impossible.

At what speed should you exercise? The best routine will incorporate slow and fast movements. In the gym, I have seen some people train very slowly, concentrating on the muscle they are working, and I have seen others move very rapidly, pumping out repetition after repetition. Since the first few reps are actually the hardest for your muscles, you should perform your movements in a guarded fashion to avoid any quick jerking or uncontrolled motions that could cause injury to the muscle. During the last few repetitions, you should try to move as fast as you can. Although these may seem harder for you because you're tired, the final repetitions are much easier for the warmed-up muscle. The fast movement has little chance of causing injury at this stage. So start out slowly and increase your speed progressively until, by the time you reach the end of your set, you're moving as rapidly as possible. You should select the number of repetitions you wish to do, but a set should *not* be terminated simply because that particular number of repetitions has been performed. Instead, complete as many repetitions in good form as you can, and then cheat with as many more repetitions as possible, stopping only when additional movement becomes impossible. If the number of repetitions performed in good form is less than the predetermined guide figure (the guide figure is usually 8 repetitions), then use the same amount of resistance for the next workout. However, if you *can* perform all the repetitions in good form, then the weight should be increased in the next workout.

If you are interested in seeing your muscles get far better than they are now, then you should constantly strive to increase the performance and the resistance, as well as increasing the repetitions, while keeping in mind the guide figure mentioned above. You should use good form and try to envision your growth as you perform each movement. This is known as progressive training, and it is a basic requirement of any worthwhile improvement you hope to achieve. Do not fall into the habit of selecting a given amount of weight or resistance and then performing a certain amount of repetitions, stopping short of complete exertion or failure. If you do this, you're only working the existing level of development you have already accomplished, and no matter how much of it you do, it will never ever produce anything in the way of the properly progressive growth stimulus you're looking for.

Proper stimulation is an important factor in muscle growth. There is a very delicate balance between good training and maximum stimulation. You have to push yourself just enough to work all the muscle fibers to the point of stress. If you have a low tolerance to pain, you must push beyond it to achieve positive gains. A muscle should be tired, pumped, and hurt a bit. See how much exercise a muscle group can take before you get exhausted, and plan your workouts accordingly. If you follow the gradient steps in the Atomic Fitness System, you will be able to handle anything.

Unless an individual's general fitness level is excellent, he or she will achieve less than his or her optimum level during Atomic Fitness training. Therefore, the first levels of exercise are aimed at achieving optimum fitness levels—at building a solid foundation for the real work to follow. That will be the exercise you need to create the ultimate physique.

At the beginning, I recommend spending about 20 percent of your time on muscle building, and the other 80 percent working to create an overall top condition for the body. This will involve the heart, lungs, and other organs, as well as the joints, ligaments, muscles, and support structure, with particular attention paid to injured or weak areas.

The volume of exercise is important; the volume of time spent training is not. In the Atomic Fitness System, emphasis is placed on a large variety of exercises and different joint movements. In the beginning, most of the exercises are to be done with dumbbells to help develop joints and stabilizer muscles. As you progress, barbells and exercise machines will be added, and further down the road you'll add some strength training into the routine to prevent injury. A strong muscle spares the tendon, which usually takes the brunt of the force. One property of muscle is that it stretches, whereas tendons and ligaments do not.

The first level of training, the preparatory stage, which is contingent on an individual's current level of fitness, should not last more than three months. In the next stage, generalized conditioning continues, and a more intense training period begins. The volume of exercise increases, with a decrease in exercise time. This will increase the intensity and the complexity of the muscle exercised. The routines are demanding, but the results are colossal. Without the proper completion of the first phase, however, the trainee will not be able to successfully move into phase two and above, so be careful to never move on to another level until you have mastered the previous one.

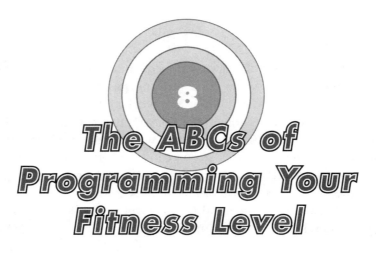

The ABCs of Programming Your Fitness Level

I f you've read everything up to this point, you should have a complete understanding of what you're about to do. Congratulations. You're about to embark on a great experience. I'm sure you have now discovered you have phenomenal potential and are ready to unleash it. As you get started, you should begin to feel better and see results in less than a week. You have the power to change your body and you will.

First, you must determine your current level of fitness and what routine is appropriate for you to begin with. The routines in this chapter include:

- The Preconditioning Routine
- Beginning Routine I
- Beginning Routine II
- Intermediate Routine I
- Intermediate Routine II
- Advanced Routine I
- Advanced Routine II

The Preconditioning Routine should be chosen if you have never had a formal exercise routine, have not worked out consistently in the past, have experienced a serious injury, or are currently recovering from an injury or pain in the body. You may also choose this routine if you're a beginner and simply don't know where to start. It is always better to begin with a simpler routine and advance from there, rather than start at a more difficult level and risk strain or injury.

Beginning Routines I and II are for those who participate in some form of aerobic activity for at least thirty minutes, at least two days a week, and are not currently injured or recovering from an injury. These routines are also appropriate for introducing those who have little or no experience with free weights to the proper techniques of training with dumbbells.

Intermediate Routines I and II are for those who engage in three or more days a week of aerobic activity and have a solid background in weight lifting. These routines require the use of exercise machinery and are especially appropriate for those training in a gym.

Advanced Routines I and II are for those who are currently in superior physical condition, and consistently participate in three or more days of aerobic activity for a minimum of thirty minutes per session. A solid background in weight training and proper form is required. These routines should not be attempted by anyone who has not mastered Intermediate Routines I and II, and are not recommended as a starting point for anyone in less than exceptional physical condition with extensive weight-training experience.

These routines are provided to help you plan an effective practice that will produce results while adapting to your individual schedule. Choose the one you feel best suits your lifestyle and available training time.

Note: *Before beginning this, or any exercise regimen, it is important to consult your physician.*

TRAINING SCHEDULES

In doing the Atomic Fitness routines, you can utilize the following training schedules. Your schedule should be based on a realistic evaluation of available training time. First, choose any one of the following routines:

1. *Total body workouts.* Train all body parts in one workout. Repeat this routine one to three times a week, making sure you have at least one day of rest in between.

2. *Large split routines.* Train at least three body parts each workout. Train back, chest, and shoulder one day, followed by abdominals, biceps, legs, and triceps the next. Then take one or two days off and repeat.

3. *Small split routines.* Train two body parts each workout. For example, train chest and shoulders one day, followed by back and triceps the second day, and biceps and legs the third day. Take one or two days off and repeat the cycle.

4. *Preconditioning routines.* All preconditioning routines require ten straight days of workouts, followed by three days of rest.

Then, fit your selection above to the schedule below that best suits your lifestyle. Keep in mind that recent medical research supports the fact that increased muscle mass is accomplished most effectively when muscles are exercised to exhaustion. This creates a condition known as hypoxia—a lack of oxygen in the body tissue. It is theorized that the body responds to this imbalance by recruiting progenitor cells from the bone marrow and blood-stream to help repair the damaged area. This is the reason why the old adage or myth of overtraining does not exist. In our opinion, you cannot overtrain. This myth has no place in modern exercise. With that said, feel free to apply any of the following training schedules to whatever routine suits you. Your choices include:

Choice A. 2 days a week

Choice B. 3 days a week

Choice C. 3 days on, 2 days off; repeat

Medical Information

Please answer "yes" or "no" to the following questions:

■ Have you been diagnosed with a heart condition?

■ Do you have any health problems that cause you pain or create limitations that must be addressed when developing an exercise program, such as arthritis, back problems, diabetes, high blood pressure, or a sports injury?

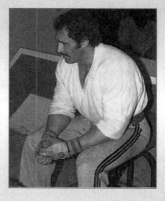

■ Are you currently pregnant, or have you given birth within the last six months?

■ Have you recently had surgery or sustained an injury?

■ Do you lose balance or consciousness when participating in physical activities?

If you have answered "yes" to any of the above questions, seek medical advice before beginning this, or any, exercise program.

Choice D. 3 days on, 1 day off, 3 days on, 2 days off; repeat

Choice E. 3 days on, 1 day off; repeat

Choice F. 4 days on, 1 day off, 1 day on, 1 day off; repeat

Choice G. 4 days on, 2 days off; repeat

Choice H. 4 days on, 1 day off; repeat

Choice I. 6 days on, 1 day off; repeat

Choice J. 6 days on, 2 days off; repeat

Choice K. 10 days on, 3 days off; repeat

If choosing "Choice C," for example, you might train on Saturday, Sunday, and Monday. Take Tuesday off and begin your training again on Wednesday, Thursday, and Friday. Take Saturday off and continue the pattern.

Note: Aerobics will be incorporated into the schedule you choose and will be performed during your training days.

PRECONDITIONING ROUTINE

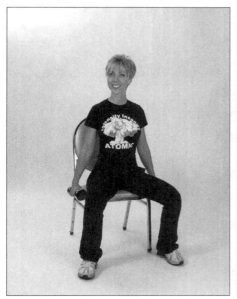
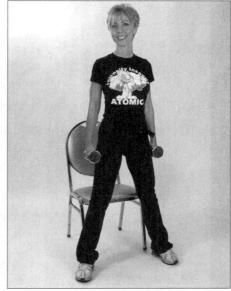

Exercise: Chair squats (sit and rise to your feet, arms at sides)
Targeted Body Part: Legs, hips, and butt

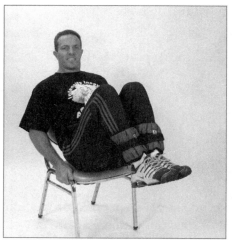 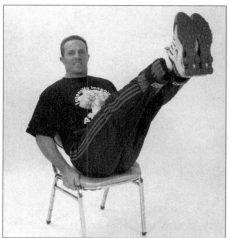

Exercise: Leg extensions in chair (bring knees into chest and then straighten)
Targeted Body Part: Legs, hips, and butt

Guidelines for Workout Routines

When performing the routines, it is important to follow these guidelines:

- Have a log book with you.
- Wear lightweight, loose-fitting clothes, and have a water bottle handy.
- Have your Atomic Fitness workout ready.
- Pick resistance for each movement and record it.
- Perform each rep slowly at first, using a full range of motion, then gradually pick up speed.
- Breathe normally and rhythmically.
- Rest for as short a period as possible between sets, only to normalize your breathing. If your breathing is okay, you don't need to rest.
- Set your goal in your mind. Put your purpose out there in the future.
- Write down how long your training took from start to finish. Record all pertinent information regarding that training session.

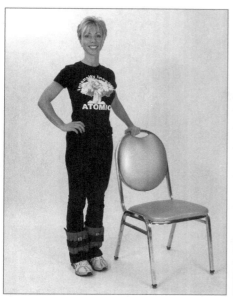
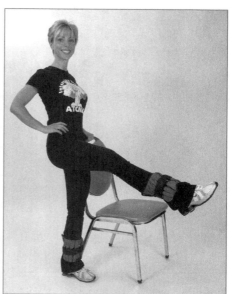
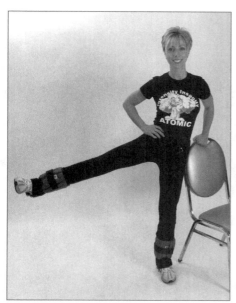
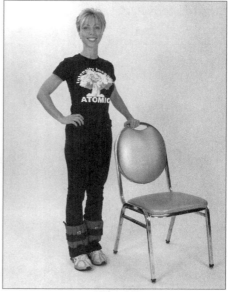

Exercise: Standing front/side leg lifts (hold on to the back of a chair, raise one leg to the front, return, then raise to the side)

Targeted Body Part: Legs, hips, and butt

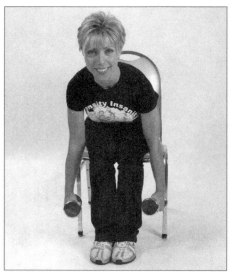
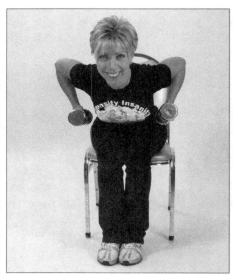

Exercise: Seated rows (hold arms straight out in front of you, palms facing each other; pull hands to your chest bringing elbows back)
Targeted Body Part: Back

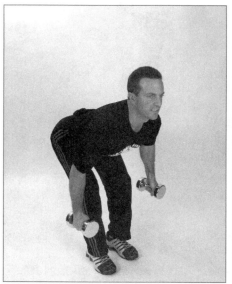
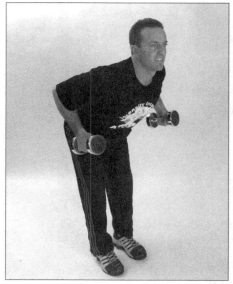

Exercise: Bent-over dumbbell rows (standing, bent at the waist, hold arms straight out with your palms facing each other; pull hands to your chest bringing your elbows back)
Targeted Body Part: Back

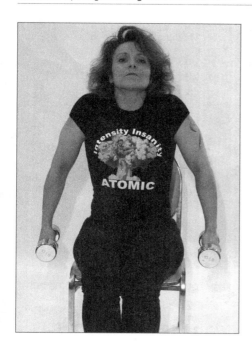

Exercise: Seated shoulder shrugs (with your arms straight down at your sides, shrug your shoulders up toward your ears)

Targeted Body Part: Back

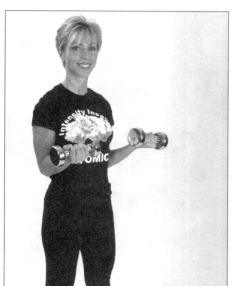
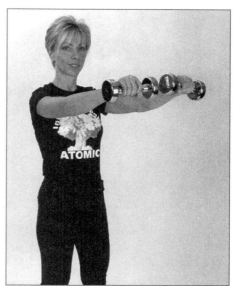

Exercise: Chest press (bent elbows out, bring fists to sides of chest, and push arms straight out in front of you)

Targeted Body Part: Chest

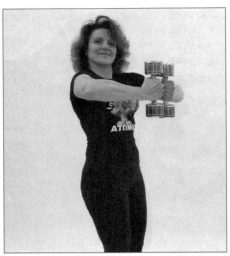 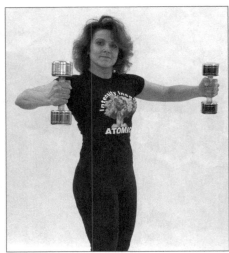

Exercise: Standing flyes (bend elbows out, bring fists together in front of chest, and pull apart and back)
Targeted Body Part: Chest

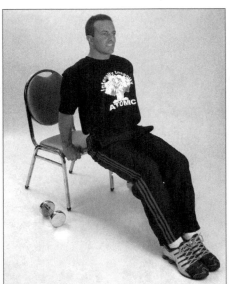 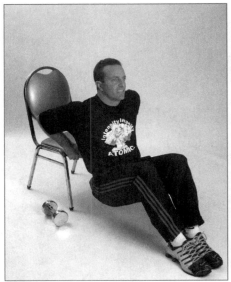

Exercise: Bench/chair dips (using a bench or a chair, lean slightly forward, grasp the edge of the bench or chair, and lift your upper torso until your elbows are straight; lower yourself back down)
Targeted Body Part: Chest

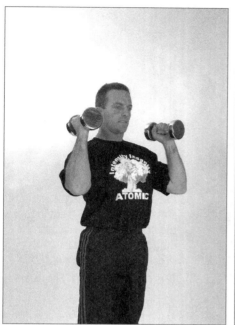 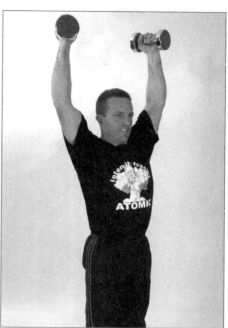

Exercise: Military press (bend arms up with fists at shoulders, push up, and bring back down)
Targeted Body Part: Shoulders

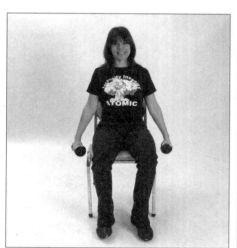 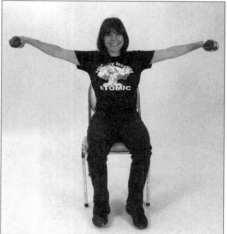

Exercise: Lateral raises (arms straight down at your sides, raise up to shoulder level and lower back down)
Targeted Body Part: Shoulders

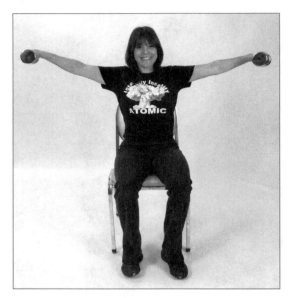

Exercise: Shoulder rotations (hold arms out at sides perpendicular to the body; rotate in a circular motion forming smaller to larger circles)
Targeted Body Part: Shoulders

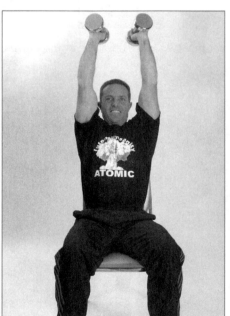 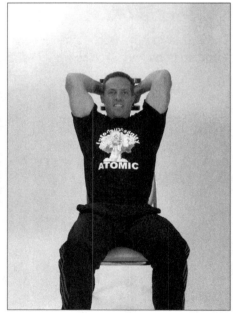

Exercise: Overhead dumbbell triceps extension (raise arms above your head, reaching toward the ceiling with thumbs facing behind you; bend your elbows, bringing your hands down so they are touching the back of your head; return to the upright position)
Targeted Body Part: Arms (triceps)

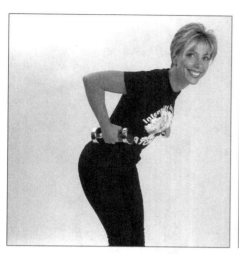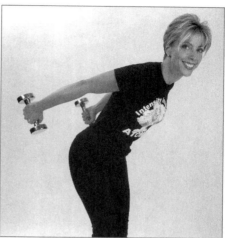

Exercise: Tricep kickbacks (using the back of a chair for support if necessary, bend over so that your upper body is parallel to the floor; raise the arm that is not supporting you so it is level with your back and your hand is pointing behind you; bend your elbow, lowering hand to the floor and return again to the straight-arm position)

Targeted Body Part: Arms (triceps)

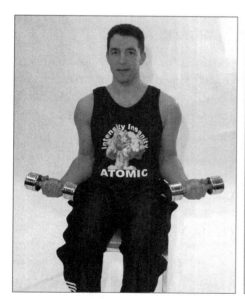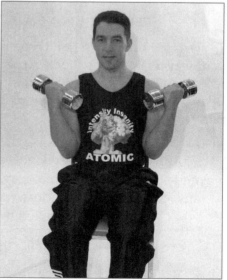

Exercise: Dumbbell curls (with your arms down at your sides and palms facing up, bend at the elbows, bringing hands up toward the shoulders, and return back down)

Targeted Body Part: Arms (biceps)

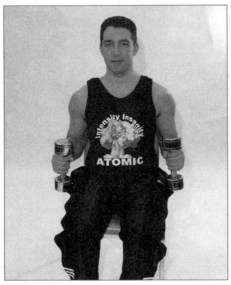 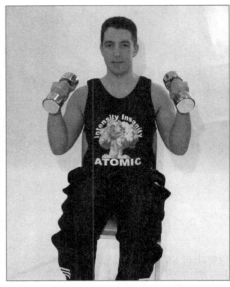

Exercise: Zottman curls (with your palms facing in, repeat the same movement as described for dumbbell curls on page 79)
Targeted Body Part: Arms (biceps)

PRECONDITIONING ROUTINE SETS/REPS

To start, perform one set of 5 repetitions (reps) for each exercise, working your way up to 25 reps. Add a rep or two each day as you feel stronger.

Aerobics: Walking or stationary bike—Start with 5 minutes and work up to 30 minutes at a nice, slow pace. Stay within 60 percent of your heart rate.

Note: Aerobics are done independently of the routines and are aimed at burning fat, not building muscle, but they may accompany any routine. You can choose whatever aerobic activity you like— the above are merely suggestions.

BEGINNING ROUTINE I

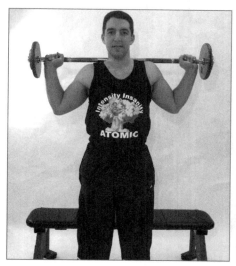 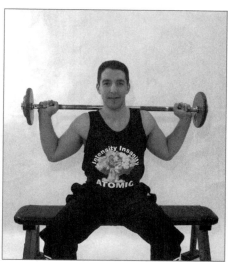

Exercise: Bench squat (with barbell)
Targeted Body Part: Upper legs and hips

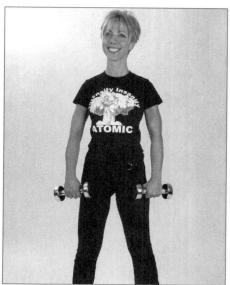 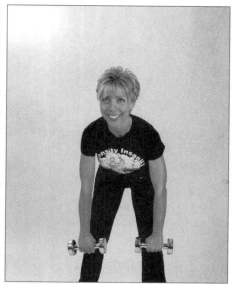

Exercise: Partial dead lifts (with dumbbells)
Targeted Body Part: Legs and hips

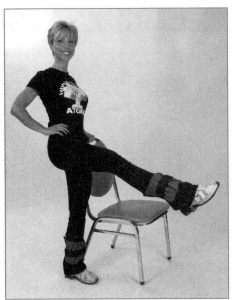
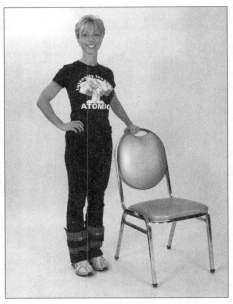

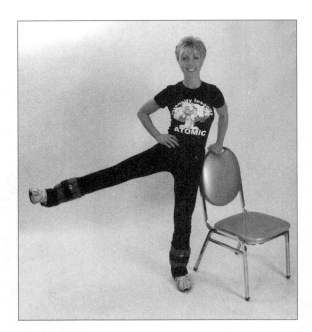

Exercise: Front/side leg lifts (with ankle weights)
Targeted Body Part: Hips

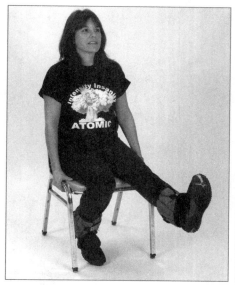 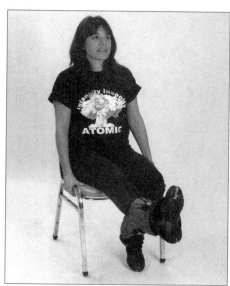

Exercise: Seated alternate leg extensions (with ankle weights)
Targeted Body Part: Lower thighs

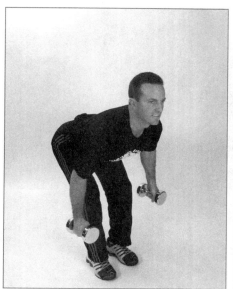 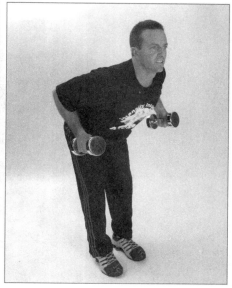

Exercise: Bent-over dumbbell row
Targeted Body Part: Back

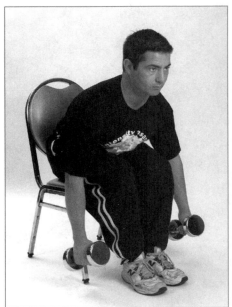
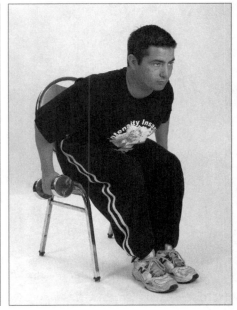
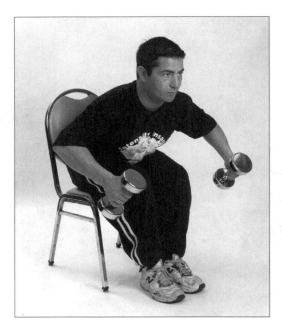

Exercise: Churns (with dumbbells)
Targeted Body Part: Back

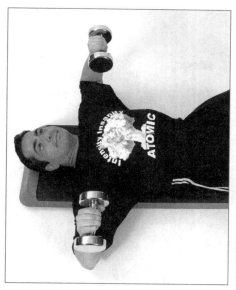
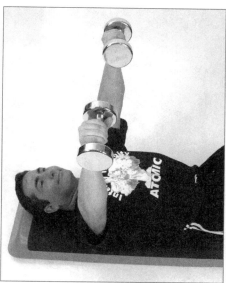

Exercise: Lying chest press (with dumbbells)
Targeted Body Part: Chest

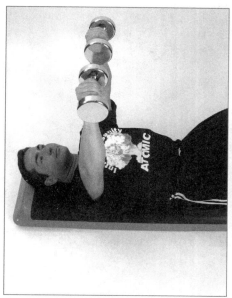
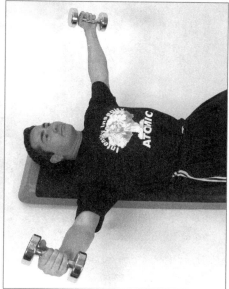

Exercise: Lying dumbbell flyes
Targeted Body Part: Chest

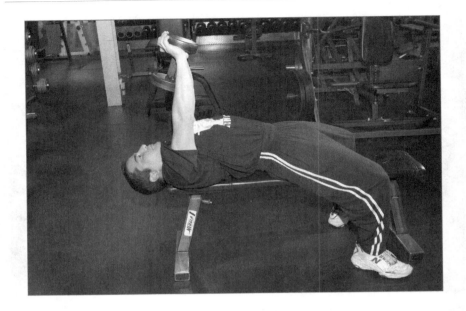

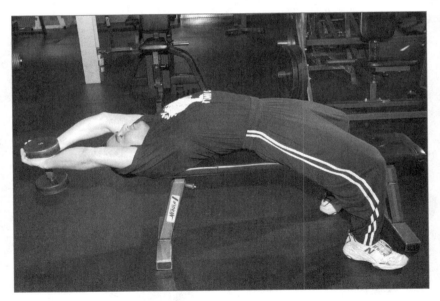

Exercise: Lying dumbbell pullovers
Targeted Body Part: Chest

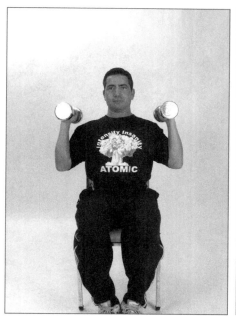 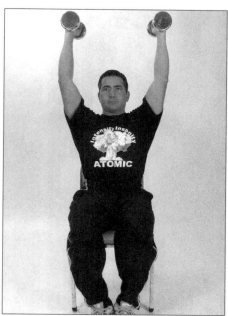

Exercise: Seated dumbbell press
Targeted Body Part: Shoulders

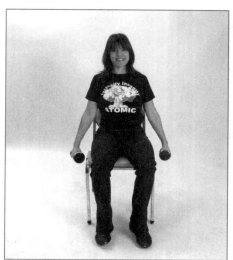 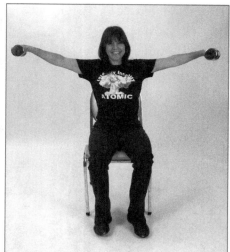

Exercise: Seated side dumbbell laterals
Targeted Body Part: Shoulders

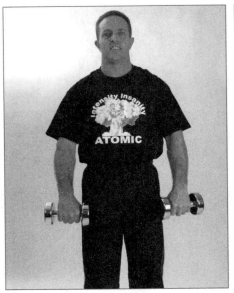 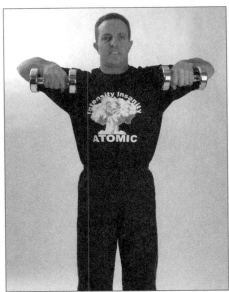

Exercise: Standing upright row
Targeted Body Part: Shoulders

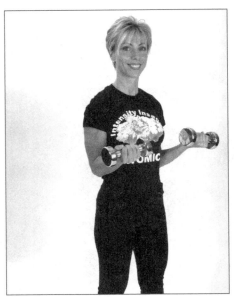 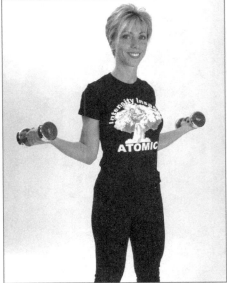

Exercise: Standing dumbbell rotators
Targeted Body Part: Shoulders/upper back

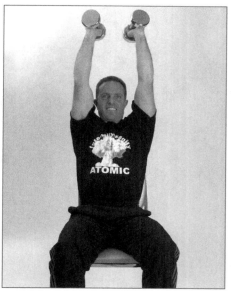 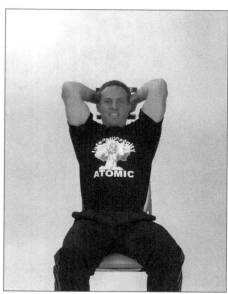

Exercise: Overhead dumbbell triceps extension
Targeted Body Part: Arms (triceps)

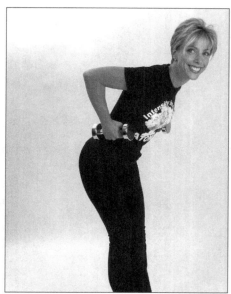 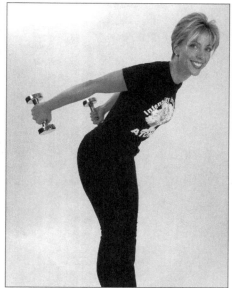

Exercise: Tricep kickbacks
Targeted Body Part: Arms (triceps)

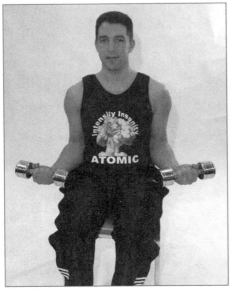 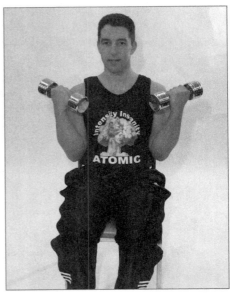

Exercise: Dumbbell curls (with palms facing up)
Targeted Body Part: Arms (biceps)

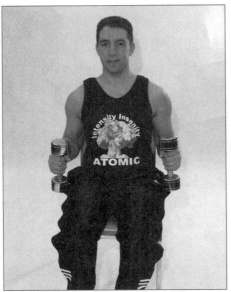 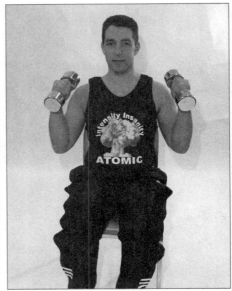

Exercise: Zottman curls (with thumbs facing up and palms facing toward each other)
Targeted Body Part: Arms (biceps)

BEGINNING ROUTINE I SETS/REPS

Begin with a single set of 25 reps for each exercise and complete the entire routine. This is one cycle. Work quickly, but maintain form. When completing one set of 25 reps becomes relatively easy, advance to two sets of 25 for each exercise. Eventually, work your way up to four sets of 25 reps for each exercise. When you're able to complete this final cycle, you're ready to move on to Beginning Routine II.

BEGINNING ROUTINE II (SUPER-SET ROUTINE)

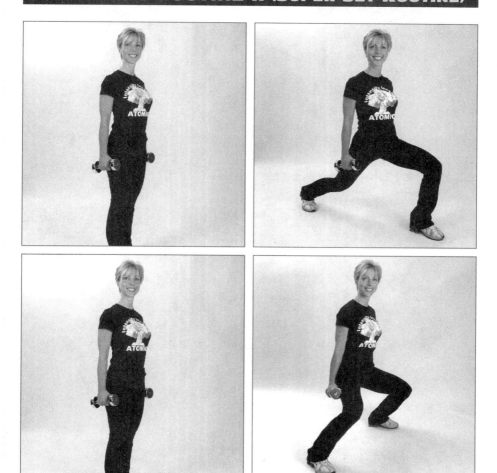

Exercise: Three-way lunge
Targeted Body Part: Upper legs and hips

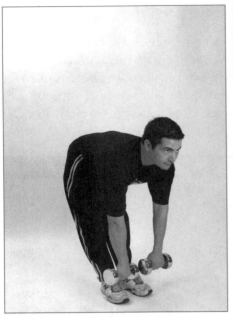 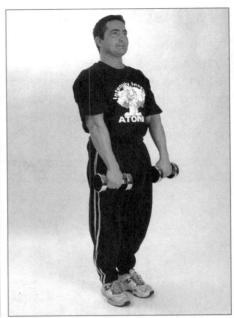

Exercise: Dead lift
Targeted Body Part: Back of legs and hips

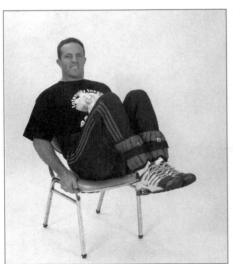 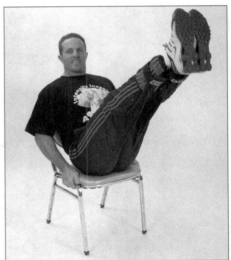

Exercise: Leg extensions in chair
Targeted Body Part: Upper thigh

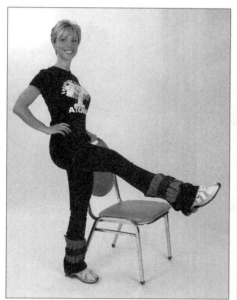
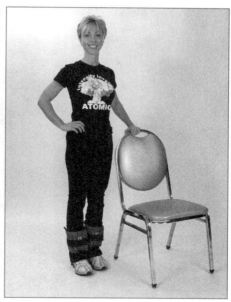
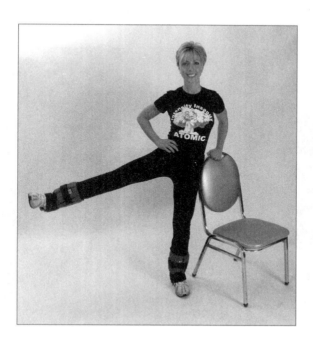

Exercise: Front/side leg lifts
Targeted Body Part: Butt and hips

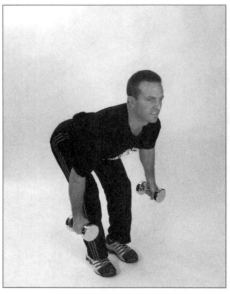 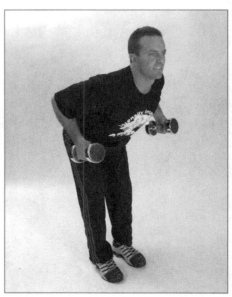

Exercise: Bent-over dumbbell row
Targeted Body Part: Back

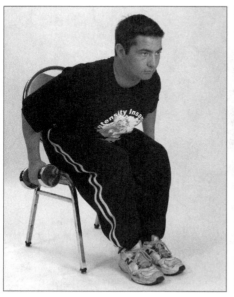 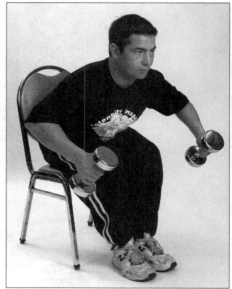

Exercise: Churns (with dumbbells)
Targeted Body Part: Back

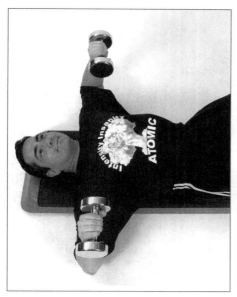 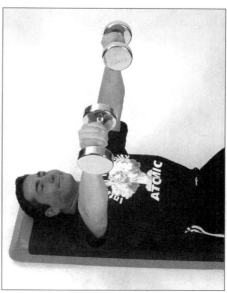

Exercise: Lying chest press (with dumbbells)
Targeted Body Part: Chest

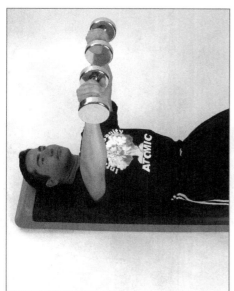 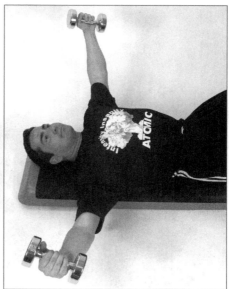

Exercise: Lying dumbbell flyes
Targeted Body Part: Chest

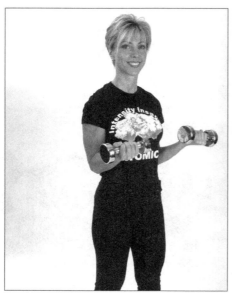 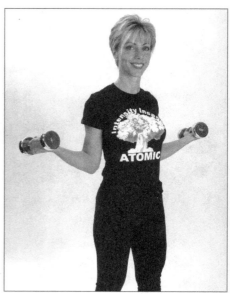

Exercise: Standing dumbbell rotators
Targeted Body Part: Shoulders/upper back

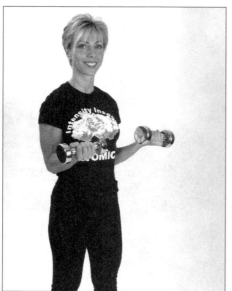 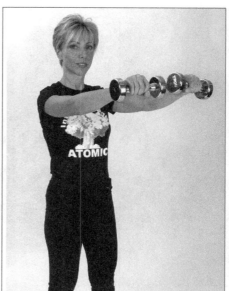

Exercise: Push-outs
Targeted Body Part: Shoulders and trapezoids

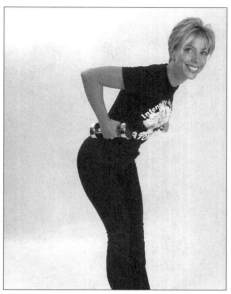 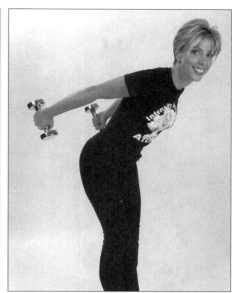

Exercise: Tricep kickbacks
Targeted Body Part: Arms (triceps)

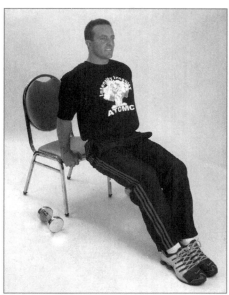 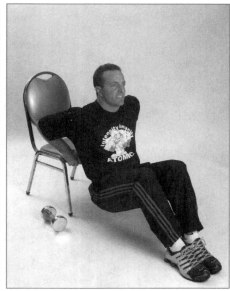

Exercise: Bench/chair dips
Targeted Body Part: Arms (triceps)

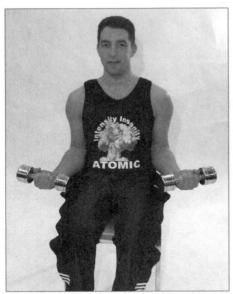 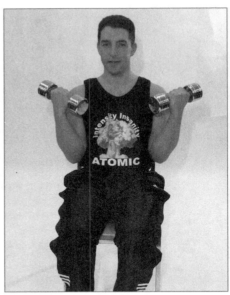

Exercise: Dumbbell curls (with palms facing up)
Targeted Body Part: Arms (biceps)

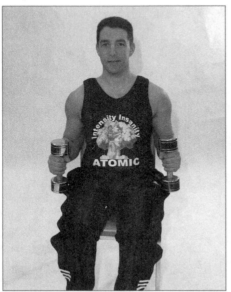 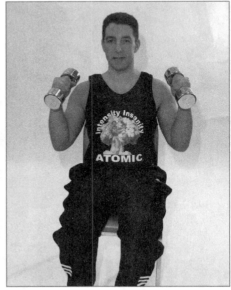

Exercise: Zottman curls
Targeted Body Part: Arms (biceps)

BEGINNING ROUTINE II SETS/REPS

This is a super-set routine, meaning that two exercises are combined for each body part. They should be performed as if they were one exercise, with little to no resting period between techniques. For example, when working the chest, perform 15 reps of presses followed immediately by 15 reps of flyes.

To begin, start with one set of 15 reps for each exercise until the entire routine is complete. When this becomes relatively easy, advance to two sets of 15 reps, and then three sets of 15 reps.

After you've mastered three sets of 15 reps, advance to two sets of 25 reps. When you've mastered this final challenge, you're ready to advance to Intermediate Routine I.

DID YOU KNOW?
Helpful Hints and Myth Busters for Training and Exercise

1. Recovery is probably the least acknowledged property of bodybuilding; yet, if you don't allow your body to recover from workouts or from everyday stress, it will eventually break down and get sick and injured, and you can forget about building muscle. If you're waking up with stiff muscles and joints, if you're feeling washed-out and fatigued, you're not building muscle. Your body is in toxic shock and cellular disrepair. However, once these toxic byproducts of exercise are removed from your system, you'll look and feel dramatically better.

2. Need a little extra boost in your workout? Try taking glycine, a potent amino acid that plays a pivotal role in energy production. Spike that glycine with NAC (N-acetylcysteine, an amino-acid building block) and get the optimum precursor to the basic structure of muscle. Both items can be easily found in any good health food or vitamin store. Try taking these before a workout and watch your power soar.

3. Abdominal work, gimmicks, classes, or anything else related to exercising the midsection will never reduce your waist size. Only a good solid diet, designed for your body will do that.

4. You can't flex fat.

5. You can't exercise off love handles.

6. You can't twist away to a smaller waistline.

7. You can't change the shape of a muscle, only its appearance, by developing surrounding muscle.

8. Heavy weights won't build size.

9. Light weights won't give you definition.

10. Resting any longer than what is required to catch your breath is useless.

11. Wide back work will not make your back wide.

12. Wide chest work will not change the shape of your chest.

13. There is no lower pectoral.

14. There is no lower bicep.

15. There is no lower anything. That includes lower abdominals. No such thing. It's all one muscle.

16. Working out at home is *not* as good as going to a gym.

17. You cannot spot-reduce body fat. Don't waste money on gimmicks.

18. You cannot swallow fitness. There is no pill. The human body was designed to move and work.

19. Full squats are primarily a butt exercise, not a thigh exercise.

20. It's not how you turn your foot that works the inner or outer calf, it's where you put the pressure on your toes: pressure on the big toe works the inner calf; pressure on the other toes works the front to outer calf.

21. The best all-around exercise for the front of the legs is the leg extension.

22. Hard cardio exercise does *not* burn fat. It burns sugar and makes your hunger go wild. You burn more fat walking than running. If you're sweating or out of breath, you're not burning fat: you're using muscle and only burning sugar.

23. If a muscle is getting fatigued, do one set working its opposing muscle, and see the effect on the original muscle—it's loaded with energy.

24. Never do the same workout within the same week. Always vary your exercises.

25. Beware—one-body-part-a-day workouts are a waste of time. Those who

appear to produce results with these workouts are using steroids, growth hormones, and insulin treatments. Don't fall for this.

26. There are no outer pectoral muscles. If you're not showing development there, then you're either not fully developed or you're just overweight.

27. Exercise *will* reduce the size of a woman's breasts.

28. The butt is all muscle. It can be developed, but you cannot exercise off the fat. That's accomplished by diet and aerobics.

29. Muscle does not turn into fat if you stop exercising. It just dissolves away.

30. You are not your body. You just live inside it, so take care of it.

31. Muscle will change only when it has to.

32. Fat is stored energy.

33. Most injuries stem from the pulling force of the opposing muscle, which is either too great or too weak. This causes a lack of balance on the muscle in front of the joint, which is too weak and the joint suffers. For example, this can occur in the knees, wrists, ankles, and back.

34. Soreness is a result of your body's inability to deliver sufficient oxygen to the exercised area.

35. Hard breathing is your body's attempt to meet oxygen demands placed on the muscle. Breathlessness is an oxygen deficit caused by the body's inability to rid itself of used oxygen in the lungs.

36. Protein drinks before or during workouts will rob the body of energy. Protein is for building, not energy.

37. The body needs carbohydrates and fluids after a workout. Eating protein right after a workout is not the way to go.

38. The advice to eat just before a workout is a myth. It takes about three hours to digest most food.

39. There are no such things as push and pull muscles. The push-pull work-out theory is worthless. *All* the muscles in the human body apply a pulling force, so forget that workout.

40. The difference between training and exercise is that when you are train-ing, you are actually flexing the muscle as you are working. During exercise, you are just trying to lift the weight or resistance for a given number of reps.

41. The lowering of resistance is what gives muscles their tone and appearance. Make sure you concentrate on that portion of any exercise.

42. To achieve maximum enlargement, the muscle must be at its maximum stretch and be moved off that stretch with a constant, steady movement, building up speed as you go.

43. There is no particular way to breathe during most exercise. Take in oxygen as you need it. Don't hold your breath. The exception to this rule is during your abdominal workout, in which you need to exhale during the contraction.

44. Trapezius muscle work is usually done with the back, not with the shoulders.

45. You must work each body part at least twice a week, or the body will believe you don't really need to change.

46. You can't be confident that all pros and trainers know how to train. The pro may have great genetics and may know how to work hard, but not necessarily work smart, and most personal trainers are sorely lacking in proper techniques.

47. Training longer and more often will never produce a champion. Intelligent training is the only way to create enough force to change.

48. Angles create and promote muscle change, and so do a variety of movements.

49. Most doctors cannot be counted on for advice on building your body. Few do it and too many are overweight and out of shape.

50. Only you can create excuses for not having the time or the energy to exercise. Take responsibility for yourself.

51. More is *not* better? Better is better.

52. The more efficient you get at an exercise, the less effective it is. So don't believe that because you're not out of breath, you're in great shape.

53. Don't be conned by fitness tips providing timesaving exercise advice for the inundated homemaker. The suggestions often include such techniques as twisting at the waist while sitting in a chair, or working the legs and butt while standing in a supermarket line, and so on. Since gains are made only when muscles undergo unusual threat, these suggestions are basically a waste of time.

54. Metabolic waste in the blood and cells is an unfortunate byproduct of hard training and may prevent you from making gains. A simple way to protect yourself is by consuming a natural botanical extract named curcuminoids. Take this neutralizing botanical and watch your muscles grow. You can get this bio-protectant from any good health food store.

55. Weight-loss organizations that emphasize some new fad diet might get you to lose weight, but a lot of that weight will be muscle, and eventually bone. Only hard exercise with intelligent eating habits will ever solve a problem of overweight.

56. One more thing—steroids. They seriously, and negatively, affect the mind and body. Trust me, you wouldn't want to go through what I did because of steroids. It wasn't pretty, so do yourself a favor and stay far away from them. (*See* Appendix C on anabolic steroids.)

INTERMEDIATE ROUTINE I

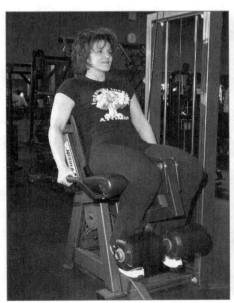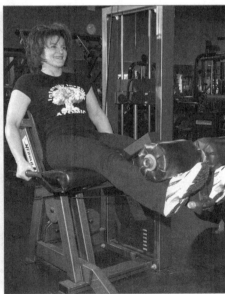

Exercise: Leg extension machine
Targeted Body Part: Legs, hips, and butt

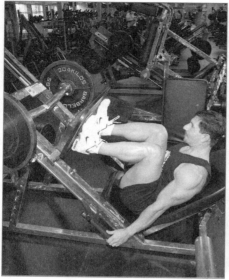 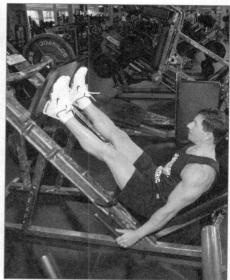

Exercise: Leg press machine
Targeted Body Part: Legs, hips, and butt

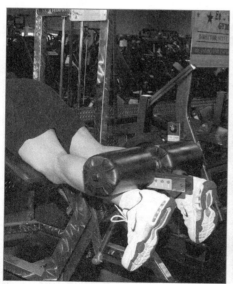 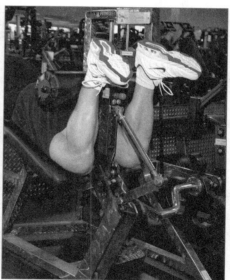

Exercise: Leg curl machine
Targeted Body Part: Legs, hips, and butt

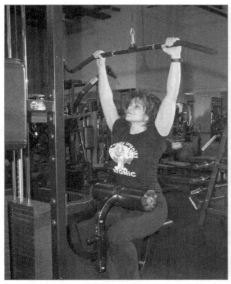
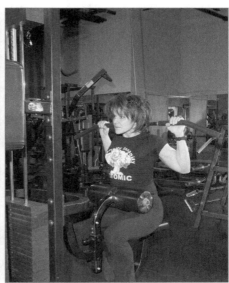

Exercise: Rear lateral machine pulldowns
Targeted Body Part: Back

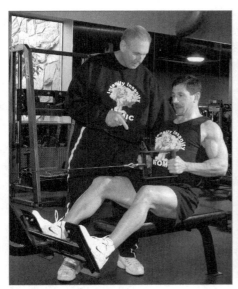
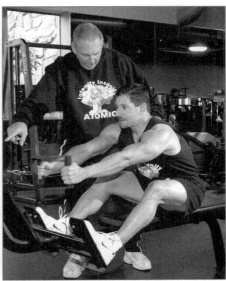

Exercise: Seated cable row
Targeted Body Part: Back

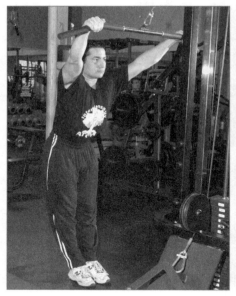 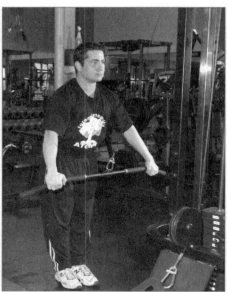

Exercise: Straight arm pulls
Targeted Body Part: Back

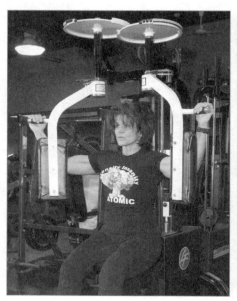 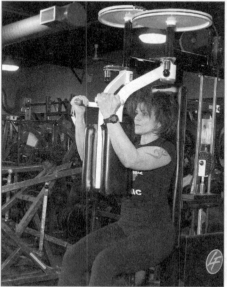

Exercise: Peck deck machine
Targeted Body Part: Chest

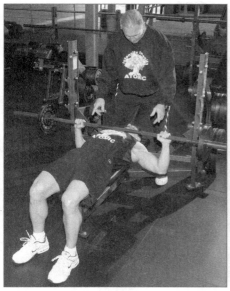 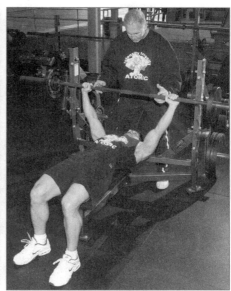

Exercise: Bench press (barbell or machine)
Targeted Body Part: Chest

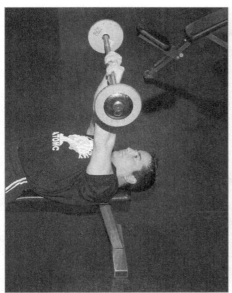 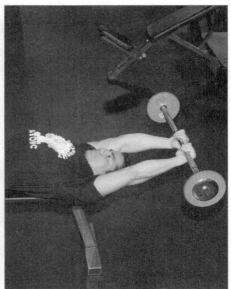

Exercise: Straight arm pullovers (with barbell)
Targeted Body Part: Chest

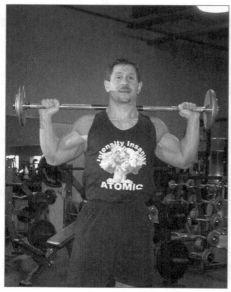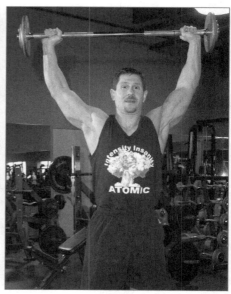

Exercise: Press behind neck (barbell or machine)
Targeted Body Part: Shoulders

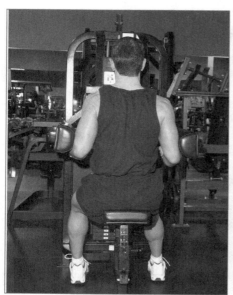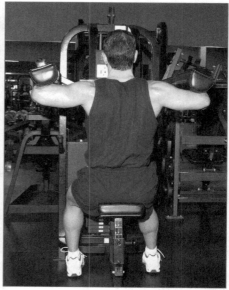

Exercise: Lateral raises
Targeted Body Part: Shoulders

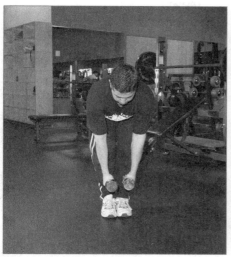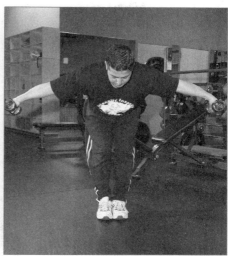

Exercise: Bent-over laterals (with dumbbells)
Targeted Body Part: Shoulders

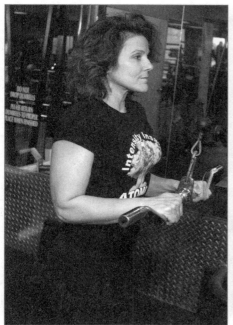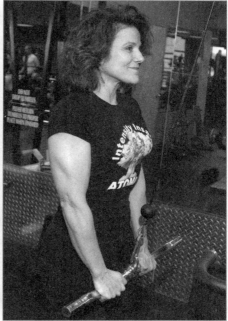

Exercise: Tricep pushdowns
Targeted Body Part: Arms (triceps)

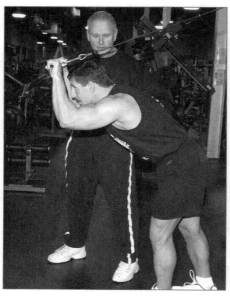 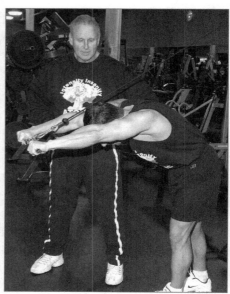

Exercise: Tricep push-outs
Targeted Body Part: Arms (triceps)

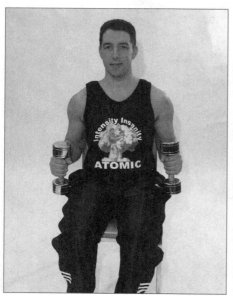 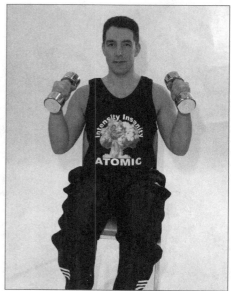

Exercise: Zottman curls (with dumbbells)
Targeted Body Part: Arms (biceps)

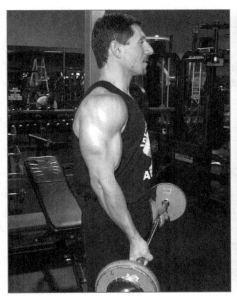 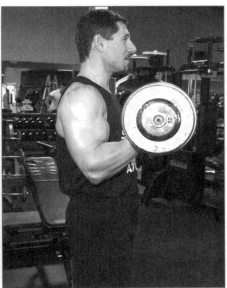

Exercise: Barbell curls
Targeted Body Part: Arms (biceps)

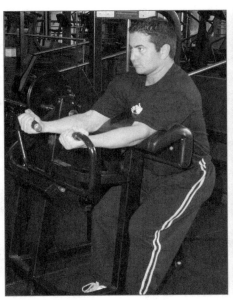 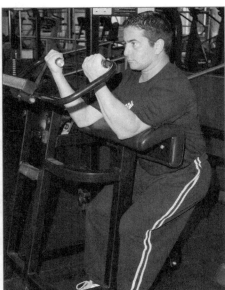

Exercise: Curl machine
Targeted Body Part: Arms (biceps)

INTERMEDIATE ROUTINE I SETS/REPS

This is a simple, progressive routine. To begin, for a total of three sets per exercise, follow the pattern of repetitions described below until you have completed the entire routine.

- First set: 25 reps
- Second set: 15 reps
- Third set: 8 reps

After you are able to successfully complete this routine one time through, increase your effort to complete the pattern of three sets twice for each exercise until the entire routine is completed. When you are able to successfully complete the pattern three times for each exercise, you are ready to advance to Intermediate Routine II.

INTERMEDIATE ROUTINE II

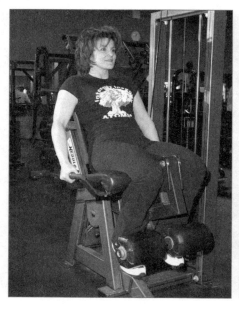 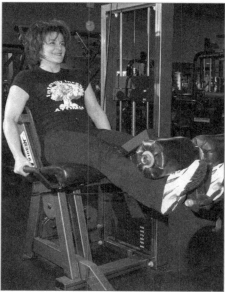

Exercise: Leg extension machine
Targeted Body Part: Legs, hips, and butt

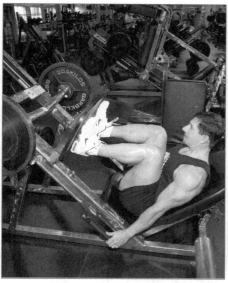 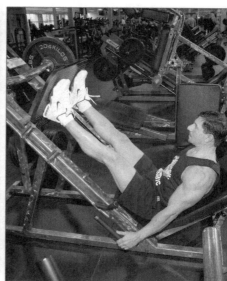

Exercise: Leg press machine
Targeted Body Part: Legs, hips, and butt

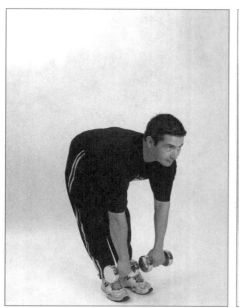 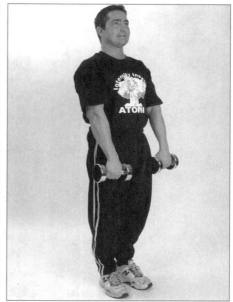

Exercise: Dead lift
Targeted Body Part: Legs, hips, and butt

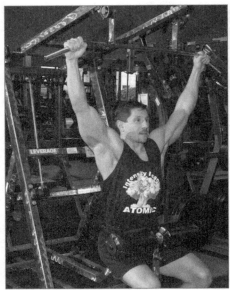 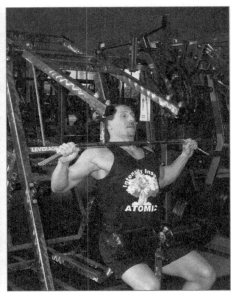

Exercise: Pull-down to front on laterals machine
Targeted Body Part: Back

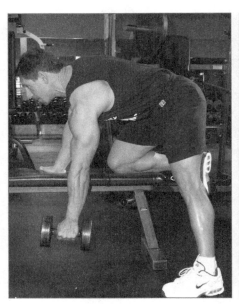 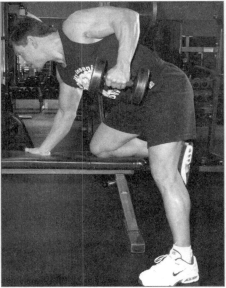

Exercise: Bent-over one-arm dumbbell rows
Targeted Body Part: Back and biceps

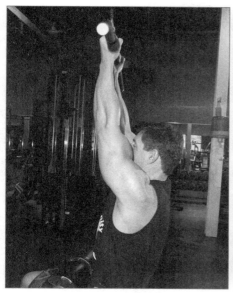 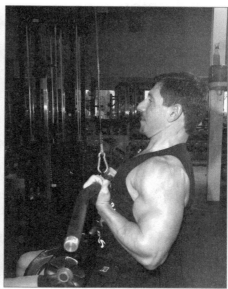

Exercise: Reverse grip pull-downs on laterals machine
Targeted Body Part: Back

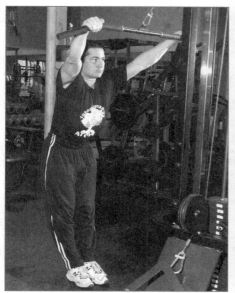 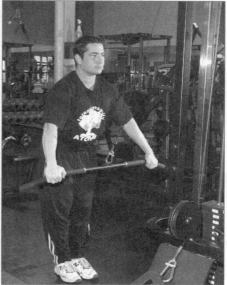

Exercise: Straight arm pulls
Targeted Body Part: Back

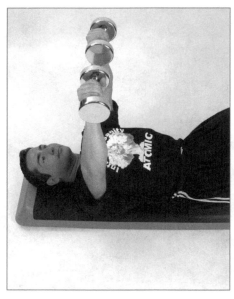
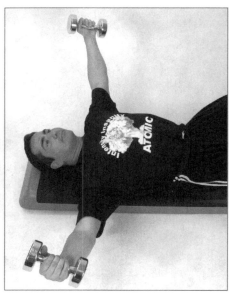

Exercise: Lying dumbbell flyes
Targeted Body Part: Chest

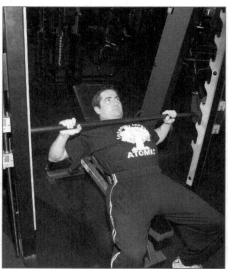
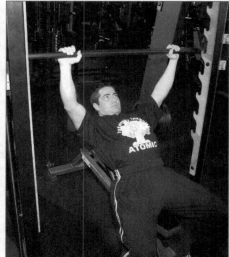

Exercise: Incline bench press on Smith machine
Targeted Body Part: Chest

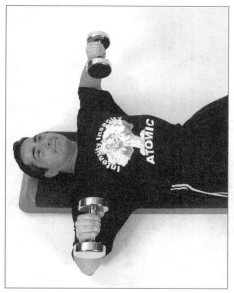 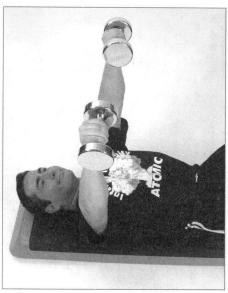

Exercise: Lying chest press (with dumbbells)
Targeted Body Part: Chest

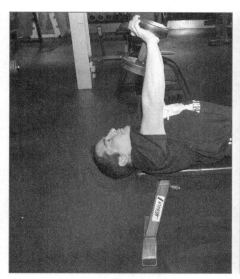 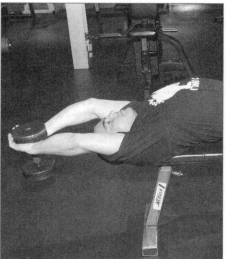

Exercise: Lying dumbbell pullovers
Targeted Body Part: Chest

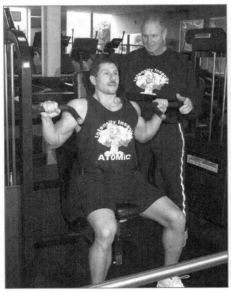 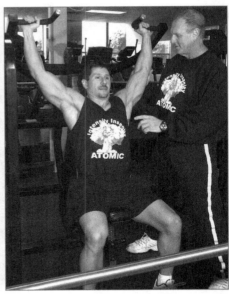

Exercise: Shoulder press machine
Targeted Body Part: Shoulders

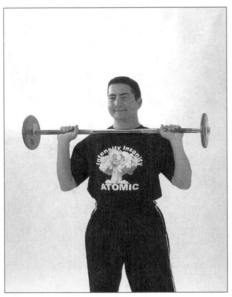 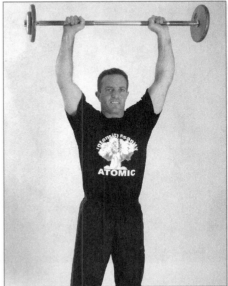

Exercise: Shoulder press with barbell
Targeted Body Part: Shoulders

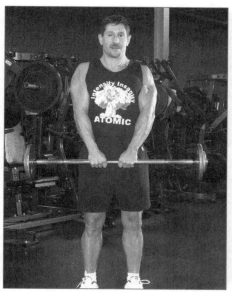 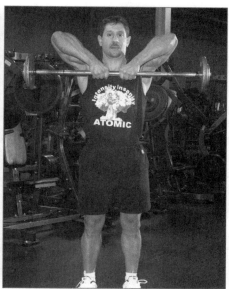

Exercise: Upright rows
Targeted Body Part: Shoulders

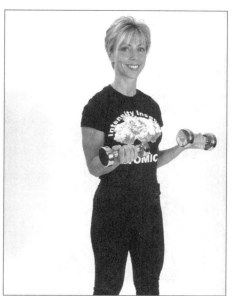 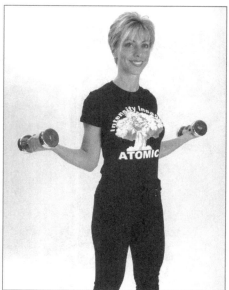

Exercise: Standing dumbbell rotators
Targeted Body Part: Shoulders/upper back

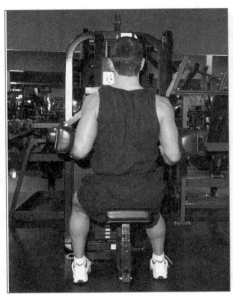 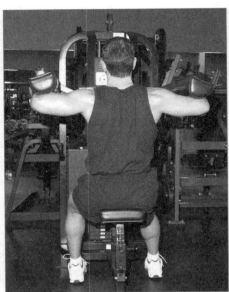

Exercise: Lateral raise machine
Targeted Body Part: Shoulders

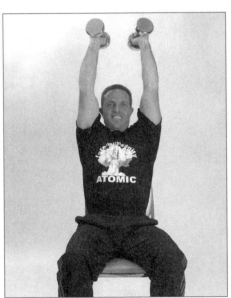 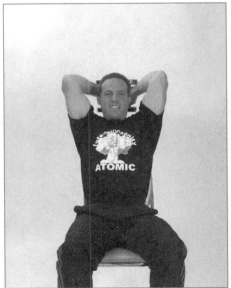

Exercise: Overhead dumbbell triceps extension
Targeted Body Part: Arms (triceps)

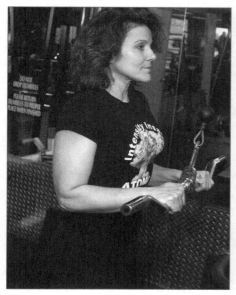
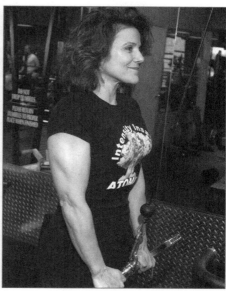

Exercise: Tricep pushdowns
Targeted Body Part: Arms (triceps)

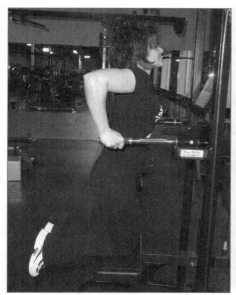
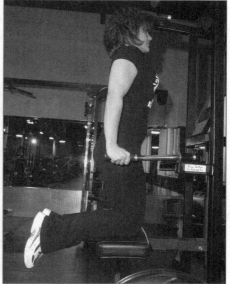

Exercise: Dips on dip machine
Targeted Body Part: Arms (triceps)

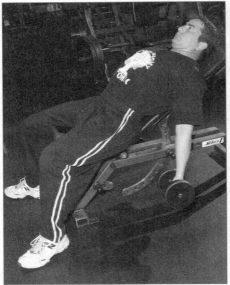 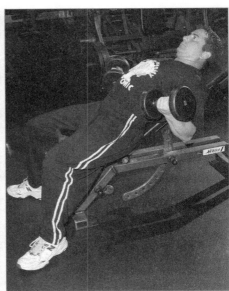

Exercise: Incline bench dumbbell curls
Targeted Body Part: Arms (biceps)

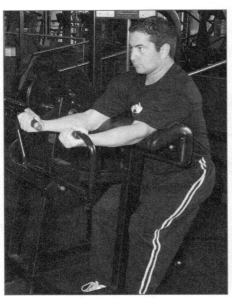 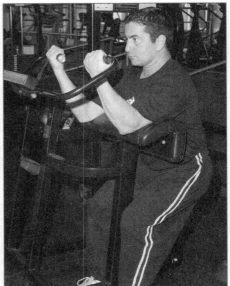

Exercise: Curl machine
Targeted Body Part: Arms (biceps)

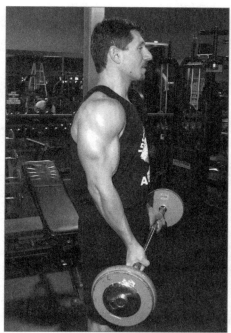 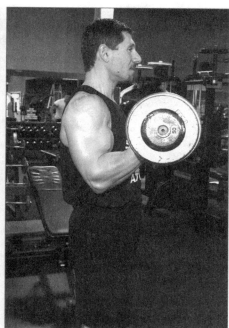

Exercise: Barbell curl
Targeted Body Part: Arms (biceps)

INTERMEDIATE ROUTINE II SETS/REPS

For this routine, you will increase weight as you decrease reps. Do each exercise in perfect form. Only use the rush factor between sets and exercise—use little or no rest.

To begin, perform two sets for each exercise. The first set will consist of 15 reps. Increase the weight and perform 8 reps for your second set.

When you're able to complete two sets for each exercise in this manner and complete the entire routine with relative ease, increase the level of difficulty by performing the entire routine of two sets twice.

When you're able to eventually complete the entire routine of two sets per exercise three consecutive times, you'll be ready to move on to Advanced Routine I.

ADVANCED ROUTINE I

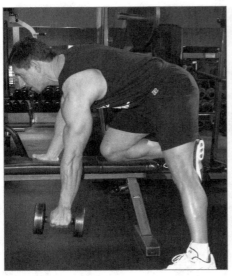 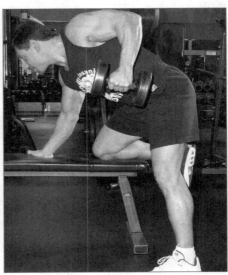

Exercise: Bent-over one-arm dumbbell rows
Targeted Body Part: Back and biceps

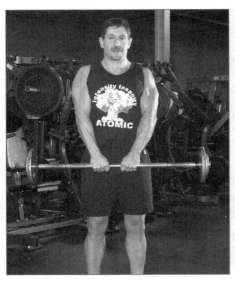 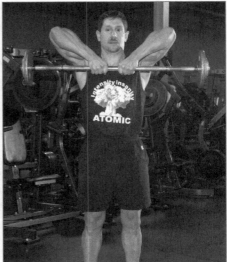

Exercise: Upright rows
Targeted Body Part: Shoulders

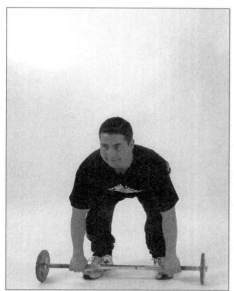
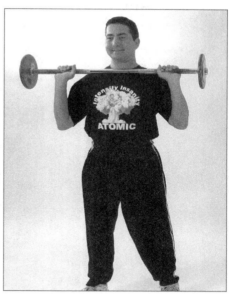

Exercise: Cleans (performed by lifting dumbbells or barbells from the floor to your shoulders)
Targeted Body Part: Total body

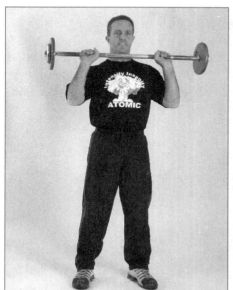
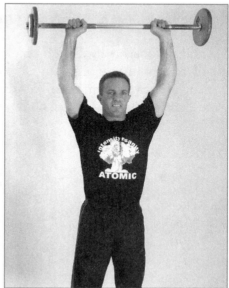

Exercise: Cleans to shoulder press (begin with Cleans, shown above)
Targeted Body Part: Shoulders

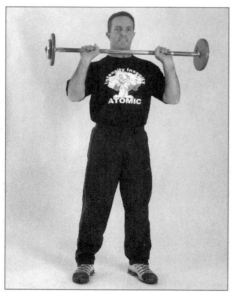
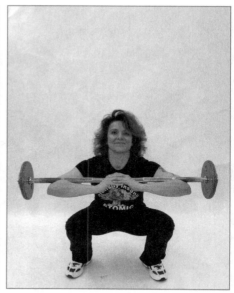

Exercise: Cleans to front squat (begin with Cleans, shown on previous page at top)
Targeted Body Part: Legs

ADVANCED ROUTINE I SETS/REPS

Maintain a consistent weight for the entire routine. Do this routine as fast as possible without stopping.

You are ready to move on to Advanced Routine II when you can complete 25 reps, one time, for each exercise.

ADVANCED ROUTINE II

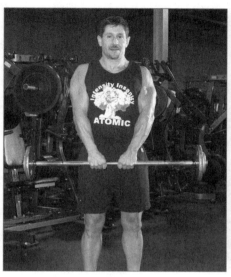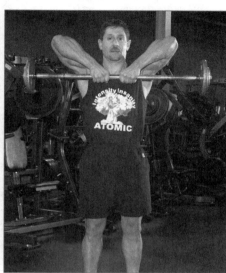

Exercise: Upright rows
Targeted Body Part: Shoulders

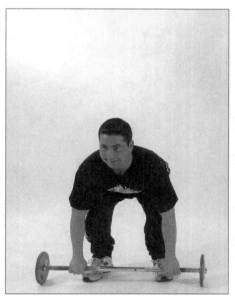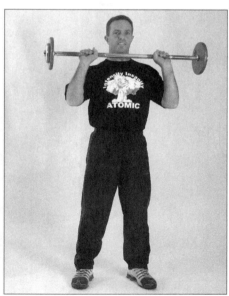

Exercise: Upright row to cleans
Targeted Body Part: Total body

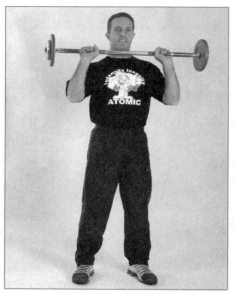 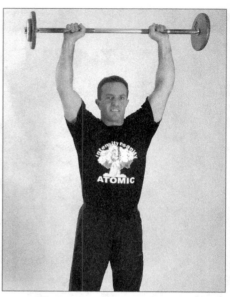

Exercise: Cleans to shoulder press (begin with Cleans, shown on page 125 at top)
Targeted Body Part: Total body

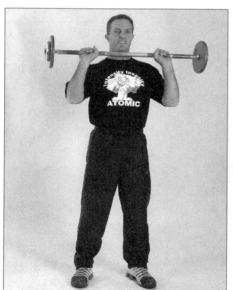 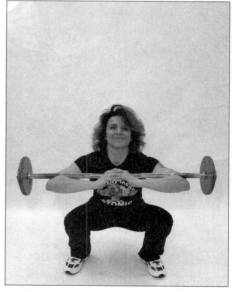

Exercise: Cleans to front squat (begin with Cleans, shown on page 125 at top)
Targeted Body Part: Total body

ADVANCED ROUTINE II SETS/REPS

Maintain a consistent weight for the entire routine. Do this routine as fast as possible, without stopping.

This is a progressive routine in which the number of reps for each exercise will increase, but the number of cleans remains constant. For example:

- 1 row: 1 clean;

- 2 rows: 1 clean;

- 3 rows: 1 clean, and so on.

When 15 repetitions have been completed for each exercise, the routine is complete.

ABDOMINALS

Trimming the waist area involves diet, fat burning, and abdominal training. While dieting alone can help reduce the waistline, it has its limitations. Dieting may take you from a big flabby stomach without muscle tone to a smaller flabby stomach without muscle tone. Either way, the area will look and feel bad. Fat-burning exercise, or aerobics, will help reduce total body fat, thereby reducing the size of the abdominals as well. However, without muscle tone, the appearance of the abdominals will not greatly improve.

One of the greatest myths in exercise is that you can work the lower and upper abdominals independent of each other. Although there appears to be an upper, middle, and lower region, abs are abs, and they are all part of one big muscle group that works to rotate the torso or trunk of the body. They cannot be segregated into sections. What causes the confusion is the amount of fat that tends to accumulate in the lower area, nature's basket. This flab convinces people that this particular region is not developing, which is simply not true. No amount of leg raises or *lower* ab exercises will improve this condition because the whole muscle, from top to bottom, contracts together. For effective abdominal training, you need to flex your entire trunk. That's it. There's no secret routine, no special equipment that will target a specific area. To get rid of that excess fat around the midsection, the only cure is fat-burning aerobics.

That said, hip flex exercises, where you lift your knees to your body as with leg raises, do serve a purpose. They create an isometric burn, that is, a muscle contraction, you will feel in your lower abdominal region. This

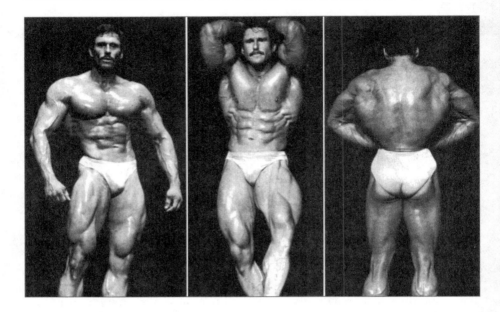

occurs because the abdominals act as a stabilizer for the psoas muscle that extends from the spine to the thigh bone. The psoas muscle does not experience a full range of motion, but it does contract isometrically, which helps its tone and strength. Hip flexor exercises also aid in strengthening the lower back area, which contributes to abdominal strength. The lower back, the psoas muscle, and the abdominals work symbiotically to stabilize the whole area. This is why I have included both hip flexor exercises and trunk exercises below.

Note: As far as oblique work is concerned, you will never exercise away love handles—never. Only a good diet and fat-burning aerobics will do that. However, if you wish to develop these oblique muscles, I've included a few good exercises to strengthen and build them. But *be cautious*—developing obliques will add to your waist size.

Abdominal Exercises

It is important to exhale during abdominal contractions. This allows your diaphragm to move out of the way so the muscles you are targeting can get the full benefit of the exercise.

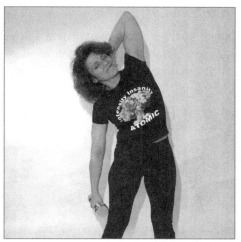

Side-bends (obliques)

With one hand behind your head and the other holding a dumbbell with your arm resting straight at your side, bend sideways bringing the dumbbell toward the floor as far as you can. Change position of hands and repeat the movement on the alternate side of the body.

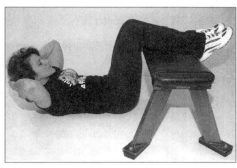

Crunches

Lying on the floor with your knees bent or your feet raised on a bench, place your hands behind your head and raise your upper body toward your knees. Do not pull yourself up with your hands, rather focus on contracting your abdominals to complete the motion. You may increase the level of difficulty by holding a weight plate behind your head for increased resistance.

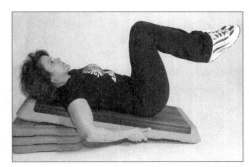

Reverse crunches

This exercise is performed in the same manner as the one above; however, this time your knees come toward your head instead of the reverse. This exercise may be intensified by using an incline board. It may also be made less difficult by resting on your elbows rather than lying flat.

Phantom twist (abdominals and obliques)

With your lower back on a padded support, such as a rolled-up towel, knees bent, and your feet secured under an immovable object, hold a weight plate at arms length directly over your face. Raise your mid to upper back off the floor about one to two inches while twisting left and right.

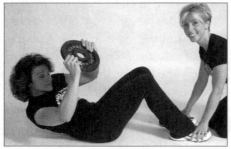 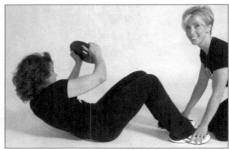

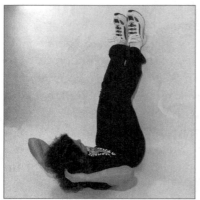

Feet against wall sit-ups

Lying flat, with your buttocks fairly close to the wall, raise your legs so they are perpendicular to your body. With knees slightly bent and feet securely planted to the wall, place your hands behind your head and raise your upper torso toward your feet. Again, it is important not to use your hands to lift your body, rather focus on flexing the abdominals and use them to perform the motion.

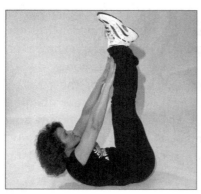

Jackknife sit-ups

Lying with your back flat on the floor, legs straight, and arms extended above your head, raise your legs while bringing your arms forward so that they're reaching for your toes. Exhale while bringing your arms and legs together and exhale on the return. Concentrate on flexing your abdominals so they are doing the work.

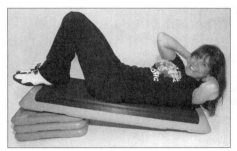

Bent-knee compound sit-ups (abdominals and obliques)

Using an incline bench with a strap for securing your feet, hook your feet under the strap, bend your knees, and place your hands behind your head with your chin resting on your chest. Twist your upper body to the right while contracting your abdominals. Make sure your lower back remains in contact with the bench. Exhale while returning to the starting position and repeat the motion on the other side.

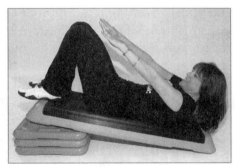

Bent-knee arms extended sit-ups

Using an incline bench with a strap for securing your feet, hook your feet under the strap, bend your knees slightly, lie flat, and extend your arms straight above your head. Lift your upper torso toward your knees while bringing your arms over your head to reach for your knees. Concentrate on flexing your abdominals so that they are performing the motion rather than your arms.

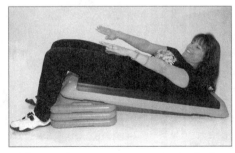

Decline arms extended compound sit-ups (abdominals and obliques)

Using a decline bench, sit on the elevated end with your feet secured beneath you. Lie back on the bench and extend your arms behind your head. Raise your torso up and over to the right until your arms are extended past your right thigh. Return to the starting position and repeat to the left.

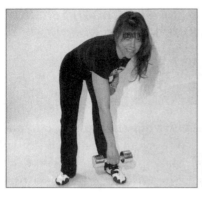

Twisting dumbbell bend to the opposite foot (obliques)

Stand straight, with your feet separated by approximately 16 to 24 inches. With a dumbbell in each hand, bend over at the waist bringing your right hand down to your left foot. Return to a standing position and repeat the movement, alternating from right to left.

Seated flat-bench leg pull-in

Sitting on the end of a flat bench, extend your legs straight out in front of you so they are parallel with the floor. Placing your hands just behind your buttocks, grasp the sides of the bench for support. Bring your knees to your chest and straighten back out. Concentrate on flexing your abdominals to perform the movement. (If this is too difficult, you may lessen the intensity by performing the movement while lying back on the bench.)

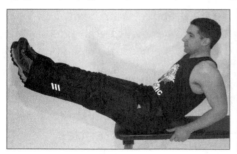
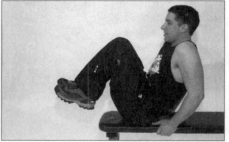

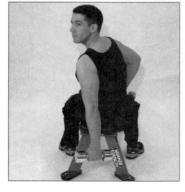

Seated dumbbell rear side bend (front and rear obliques)

Sitting on a bench with your legs to either side, position yourself so your buttocks are at the very end of the bench. Holding a dumbbell in your right hand, twist to the right and bend backward, bringing the dumbbell toward the floor. Switch hands and repeat the movement to the other side.

Standing dumbbell torso twist (obliques)

Standing straight with your legs approximately 16–24 inches apart, grasp a dumbbell with both hands and place it against your chest just below your pectorals. Keeping your back straight and your knees locked, begin twisting your upper torso to the right and left as far as you can.

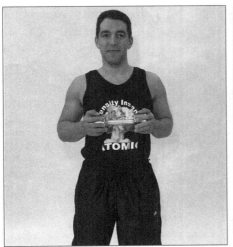
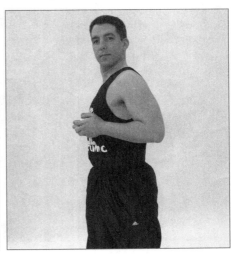

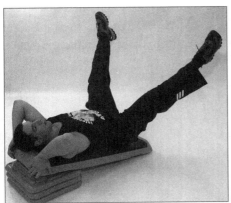

Incline V-leg raise

Using an incline bench, lie with your head at the top. Grasp the bar at the top of the bench for stability. With your legs straight and your knees locked, inhale and raise your legs up in a V position as close to a right angle with your body as possible. Return to the starting position, keeping your legs above the bench 2–3 inches, and repeat.

Dip stand leg raise

Using a dip stand, position yourself so you are facing away from the machine. Support yourself with your arms, keeping your elbows locked. Raise your legs so they are perpendicular to your body. Lower and repeat. Do not bend your knees during the movement.

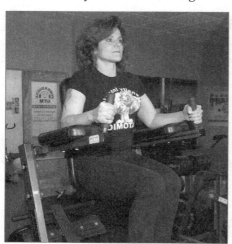 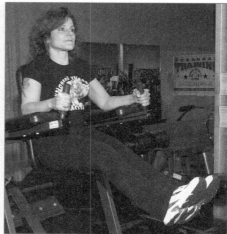

Floor Routines for Hips and Butt

The following routines for hip flexors and butt are designed to help strengthen the lower back area and thereby support abdominal strength.

Routine 1

1. While lying on a mat, position your body so you are on your side, up on one elbow. Keep your leg straight and lift it up from the side. Do 15 reps and hold for 10 seconds at the completion of the last rep.

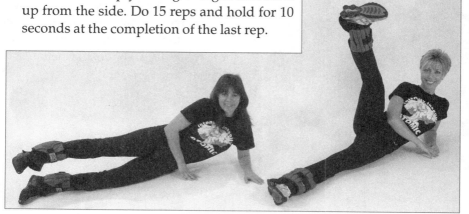

2. Next, starting with both legs straight and parallel to each other, drive your knee into your chest and back again for 15 reps.

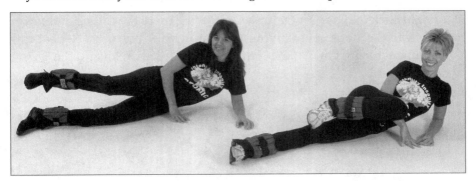

3. At your final rep, keep your knee in the bent position by your chest. Now, kick your lower leg straight out so it is perpendicular to your body. Repeat this for 15 reps.

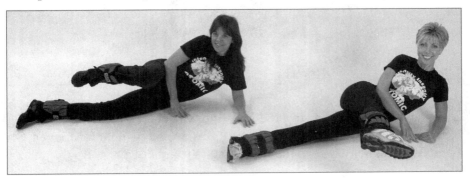

4. On the final rep, hold your leg in the perpendicular position for 10 seconds and begin raising the leg up and down, maintaining the perpendicular angle. Now, turn over onto your other side and repeat the process with the other leg.

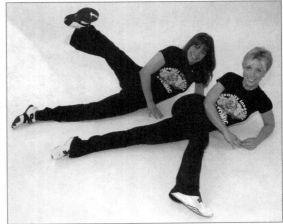

Routine 2

1. On the mat, position yourself so you are on all fours. Extend one leg straight back to the rear of your body. Lift leg up to the ceiling and lower it back to the floor, maintaining tension in your buttocks. Repeat this movement for 15 reps. On the 15th rep, hold the leg up toward the ceiling for 10 seconds.

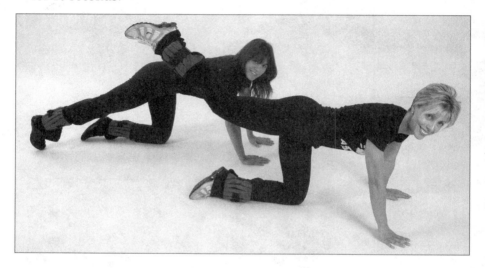

2. Using the same leg, bring the knee into the chest, then extend the leg straight back, flexing the buttocks. Repeat this movement for 15 reps. On the last rep, hold knee to the chest for 10 seconds.

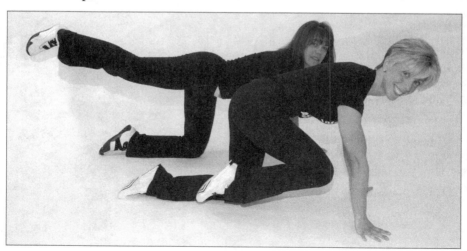

3. Keeping your leg in the bent position, lift your knee from the chest position out to the side and back again. Your leg should remain in an L shape throughout this motion.

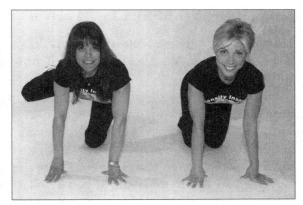

4. On the fifteenth rep, keep your leg in the raised L-shape position and begin straightening your leg without lowering it to the ground.

5. Repeat this movement for 15 reps. On the final rep, hold your leg out straight, perpendicular to the body, for 10 seconds. From this position, begin lifting your leg up and down. Re-

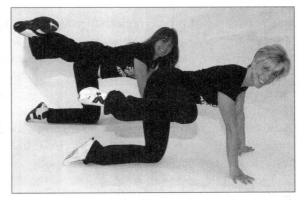

peat this movement for 15 reps.

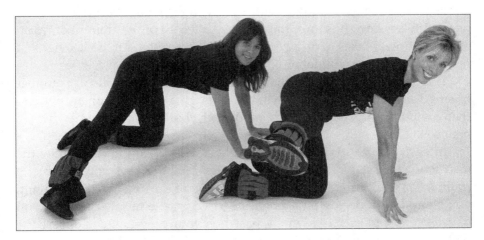

6. Switch legs and repeat the process.

THE TRAINING EFFECT—INTENSITY/INSANITY

Whatever you agree to, you will become. If you agree that you're fat, then you will be. If you disagree with a small, puny body, then it will grow big and strong.

Reality is only an agreed-upon viewpoint. Disagree and create your own reality. Disagree and be free. There are no rules, only those you create and believe to be true. If you truly believe you can't, you won't. In your training, you will come up against obstacles; you can overcome them. To do so, you must not agree with them. The system of Intensity/Insanity will only produce optimum results if you allow it to. All of life has barriers. In your training, the only real barrier is you and your willingness to confront that which seems impossible. What you really have to comprehend is that you're capable of much more than you believe you are, and that your body is set up to convince you otherwise.

I have developed a gradient method of training. It starts with a conditioning program and progresses to advanced levels of training. At each level, you will be tested. As you progress, your ability to confront exercise, as well as life, will increase.

After you've successfully gone through the beginner to advanced routines, you'll be ready for the Intensity/Insanity routines. The purpose of this system is to shock the muscles into growth, and the following routines are designed to do just that. Again, they begin with the conditioning routines and progress to the more advanced routines. The most effective way to apply the Intensity/Insanity methods would be on a gradient—you should not advance to the harder workouts until you have mastered the previous ones with certainty. It is important to keep a record of the amount of resistance and time it takes to do a routine. The goal is always to go heavier and faster, but within the guidelines of correct form.

It should be noted that, although I don't prescribe a particular number of reps, I agree with Arthur Jones of Nautilus fame who recommends no less than 8 and no more than 20. You should reach absolute failure somewhere in between.

Intensity/Insanity is designed for easy application if you follow the instructions. First, based on your schedule, pick the days you are able to train. After you've made a realistic evaluation of the time you can commit, you should then decide on a program based on the number of days you have available to exercise. Finally, based on your program, you choose the body part(s) you wish to train. For example, if you only have two days to train, you might want to consider a body split, such as the following:

- Tuesday—chest, back, and shoulders
- Thursday—arms and legs

If you have three days to train, you might want to consider training two body parts each day. As with all Atomic Fitness routines, the training schedules described earlier in this chapter are useful for planning an effective strategy adapted to your individual scheduling requirements.

Note: No exercise routine should be undertaken before consulting your physician.

ADVANCED ATOMIC FITNESS INTENSITY/ INSANITY ROUTINES

If you find you are having difficulty overcoming a plateau, or you have stalled in either fat burning or muscle building, you have reached a metabolic equilibrium. These metabolism-enhancing routines are designed to enable you to break through this barrier and upgrade your metabolism in order to achieve higher levels of fitness and muscle mass.

All Intensity/Insanity routines are prorated and have been tested thoroughly for their degree of difficulty. The levels range from 1, the least difficult, to 10, extremely difficult. Whichever of the following routines you choose (I use them all), your results will be phenomenal. Nothing you have ever tried can equal the gains you will realize after you have done some of these incredible routines. Good luck and dare to be great.

Straight Sets (1)

Do a given number of reps per exercise. For example, one set of 10.

Halves (1)

Perform half the movement of an exercise (this is called a half rep), followed by one full movement of the exercise (a full rep). This double action is considered one complete rep. Repeat until you've accomplished the desired number of repetitions.

Halves and a Full (1)

Do a full rep followed by a half rep. This action is considered one complete rep. Repeat until you've accomplished the desired number of repetitions.

Additional Techniques and Set Varieties

The following techniques and set varieties can be applied to any of the Intensity/Insanity routines.

Angular movements

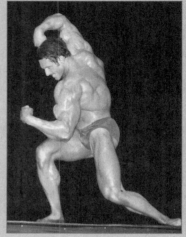

• **Chest.** When working the chest, apply force with each hand toward the center of your body and back.

• **Back.** When working the back, apply force with each hand away from the center of your body.

• **Shoulders.** When working the shoulders, apply force with each hand toward the center of your body.

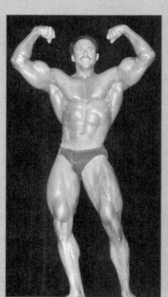

Standard set—performing any one exercise for a certain number of repetitions before moving on to the next exercise.

Super sets—grouping any two exercises together, and moving non-stop from one machine to the next after each set.

Monster sets—grouping any three exercises together, and moving nonstop from one machine to the next after each set.

Giant sets—grouping any four exercises together, and moving nonstop from one machine to the next after each set.

Jumbo sets—grouping any five exercises together, and moving nonstop from one machine to the next after each set.

Insanity sets—grouping so many exercises together at once that the difference between reality and insanity is paper thin. But the gains achieved are phenomenal.

Progressive Halves (1)

Do a half rep and a full rep. Follow with 2 half reps and 1 full rep, then 3 half reps and 1 full rep. Continue the pattern until muscle failure occurs. Continue this pattern up to 15 halves, no more. If this number is done easily, the resistance is too low.

Pyramid Sets (2)

Do a given number of reps per exercise. Then do another set of the same exercise, but this time add weight and do fewer reps, and so on.

Double Progressive Halves (2)

Do a half rep and a full rep. Follow with 2 half reps and 2 full reps, then 3 half reps and 3 full reps. Continue the pattern until muscle failure occurs.

Varied Progressive Halves (2)

Do 2 half reps from the bottom and 1 half rep at the top. Follow with 3 half reps from the bottom and 2 half reps at the top. Then do 4 half reps from the bottom and 3 half reps at the top. Repeat this pattern no less than eight consecutive times.

Dead Stops (2)

The dead stop is a great mass builder because it requires the recruitment of every available muscle fiber for each rep.

From the starting position (for example, standing), lift the weight and put it down completely, leaving no tension on the muscle. Pause for a count and repeat for designated number of reps.

Stop and Go from the Top (2)

On the way up, lift the weight and stop halfway to the top. Pause for a count and finish the rep. Repeat.

Stop and Go from the Bottom (2)

Begin by lifting the weight to the top. Pause for a count. On the way down, stop at the halfway point and pause for a count before returning the weight to the bottom.

Reverse Varied Progressive Halves (3)

Do 1 half rep from the bottom and 2 half reps at the top. Follow with 2 half reps from the bottom and 3 half reps at the top. Then do 3 half reps from the bottom and 4 half reps at the top. Repeat this pattern no less than eight consecutive times.

Digressive Sets—Strip Sets (3)

Start with the heaviest amount of weight possible. Work to muscle failure and strip some of the weight off. Work to muscle failure. Keep stripping weight off and repeat each time to muscle failure.

Push-In/Pull-Out (3)

On all pressing-type movements for shoulders and chest (such as the chest press) and pulling-type movements for the back, lift the weight approximately 1 inch and apply an inward force as you raise the weights, pushing your hands together and flexing as hard as you can for a count of three. Continue pushing together as you raise the weights to the top. On the return, apply the opposing force, pulling the weights apart as hard as you can as you come back down.

Push-In, Applied Force (3)

On shoulder and chest movements, such as the chest press, lift the weight approximately 1 inch and apply an inward force, pushing your hands together and flexing as hard as you can for a count of three. Continue pushing together as you raise the weights to the top. Relax, and then maintain the inward force again as you lower the weight. When doing back exercises, use an applied outward force, maintaining an outward pressure on whatever bar or handle you are using.

Pull-Out/Push-In (3)

On an exercise machine, such as the chest press, lift the weight approximately 1 inch and pull your hands apart, flexing as hard as you can for a count of three. Continue pulling apart as you raise the weights to the top. On the return, apply an inward force, pushing the weights together as hard as you can.

Pull-Out/Pull-Out (3)

On an exercise machine, such as a chest press, lift the weight approximately 1 inch and pull your hands apart, flexing as hard as you can for a count of three. Continue pulling apart as you raise the weights to the top. Relax and then continue this outward force as you lower the weights back down on the return. Utilize this system on all press-type movements, and on all back exercises that involve a bar.

Minute Sets (3)

For minute sets, start the exercise at the slowest possible speed, and progressively increase it until a full contraction is obtained. You might want to try using the minute-set principle along with one of the other principles. For example, you could pump out 15 reps as fast as possible, then do a minute set of 8 reps. Another variation would be one fast, intense rep, followed by a slow-paced minute set, followed by a fast-paced minute set, followed by a slow-paced minute set, and so on.

Dynamic Tension Sets (4)

Do a rep. At the most difficult point of contraction, relax and contract the muscle several times (3–6 contractions). Repeat for the given number of reps.

Isometric Hold for 14 Seconds (4)

This exercise is designed to enhance muscle striations.

Pick an exercise and move the weight to the top. Now lower the weight to a point where the muscle is in its fullest contraction. Flex as hard as you can for 14 seconds. Repeat for the given number of reps.

Assisted Stop and Go from the Top (4)

This routine requires a training partner.

Lift the weight fully. On the return, at the height of the contraction, have your training partner apply a constant, equalizing resistance against the movement for a count of three, then let go. During this time, the trainee will push as hard as possible against the resistance.

It is critical for the training partner to use pressure equal to that of the trainee's. Too much or too little resistance will render the exercise useless.

Negatives (5)

This routine requires a training partner.

Using a heavy weight, lift the weight to the top (use a spotter if necessary). The trainee must then attempt to keep the weight at the top while the partner pulls the weight down smoothly. The trainee must fight the resistance the entire way down with everything he or she has.

Positive Holds (5)

This routine requires a training partner.

Using an exercise, such as the barbell curl, the trainee will slowly start lifting the barbell. As soon as tension is felt in the muscle, the training partner will begin applying a constant, equalizing resistance to the upward motion for a count of three and then let go. During this time, the trainee will fight against the resistance with everything he or she has.

Eights (5)

Start with a resistance with which you can perform 8 repetitions of an exercise easily and lock out (bring the weight to a rest). Add weight and perform another 8 reps. Repeat the process until you can no longer do 8 reps.

Basic Progressive Training—15-12-8-6 (5)

Choose a weight that you can perform 15 repetitions with. Add weight and do 12 reps. Add weight and do 8 reps. Continue this pattern down to 6 reps.

Cardio Sets (5)

The following routine is a total body workout, addressing abs, arms (biceps and triceps), back, chest, legs (butt, calves, hamstrings, and thighs), and shoulders. One exercise per body part, using a very light weight, should alternate with short, intense sets of cardio.

Start by exercising a body part, completing 100 reps. Sprint to a cardio machine (bicycle, elliptical, stair stepper, treadmill, or other) and work as hard as you can for 3 minutes. After 3 minutes, work a different body part for 100 reps. Sprint back to a cardio machine for another 3 minutes. Continue this pattern until you have exercised each body part.

Compound Fat-Burning Routines (5)

This technique combines two or more movements in one exercise. For example, you may combine the motion of lifting your arms for a side dumbbell raise and go directly into an overhead press. This combination would be repeated for the required number of reps. The following are good examples of compound movement sets.

Total Body

- Frog squat and curl
- Frog squat and overhead extension
- Frog squat and press
- Frog squat and push-out
- Frog squat and side lateral
- Frog squat and upright row

Frog Squat

A frog squat is performed in an upright standing position with feet separated and arms extended straight down between your legs. While holding dumbbells of an appropriate weight and maintaining a straight back, bend only your knees to lower the dumbbells toward the floor. Return to the standing position for one repetition.

Chest

- Dumbbell flye to press
- Dumbbell pullover to press
- Dumbbell pullover to press to flye

Shoulder

- Bent-over rotators to bent-over laterals
- Clean to press
- Dumbbell rotators to side laterals
- Front raise to side laterals
- Monkey lift to side laterals

Back

- Dead lift to row
- Row to bent-over lateral
- Pull-down to front; pull-down to rear

Biceps

- Dumbbell pull-ins to curl
- Standing cable curl to seated cable curl to lying cable curl
- Zottman to standard curl

Triceps

- Tricep kickback to straight-arm lift to rear
- Tricep push-down to push-outs

Eights (6)

Start with a resistance that will allow you to perform 8 repetitions of an exercise easily. With a training partner, perform the 8 reps and hold the eighth one up. While the muscle is under pressure, without locking out, have your partner add weight, and perform another 8 reps. Repeat the process until you can no longer perform any movement with the weight that has been added.

Advanced Basic Progressive Training—25-15-12-8-6 (6)

Choose a weight that you can perform 25 repetitions with. Add weight and do 15 reps. Add weight and do 12 reps. Continue this pattern down to 6 reps.

Heavy Basic Progressive Training—6-4-2 (6)

For this exercise, it is important to use the heaviest weight possible and continue to increase the weight as you decrease reps.

Up and Down Eights (7)

With a training partner or two, do 8 reps and hold the eighth one up. Have your training partner(s) add weight and do another 8 reps. Repeat the process of adding weights for a total of eight times. Then repeat the process, having your training partner(s) remove weights for eight more sets on the way down.

Slow-Motion Stop-and-Go Sets (7)

Using a moderate weight, move the resistance to the top. On the return, stop every 1 to 2 inches, moving as slowly as possible, making the weight feel extremely heavy.

Pyramid Progressives—25-15-12-8-6-4-8-4-6-8-12-15-25 (8)

Following the pattern of repetitions outlined above, choose a weight that you can perform 25 repetitions with. Add weight and do 15 reps. Continue this pattern of adding weights and decreasing repetitions until you complete the 8 repetitions at the center of the pyramid. At this point, begin to decrease the amount of weight and increase repetitions until you complete the cycle.

Pattern Routines (8)

The following is a variety of pattern routines.

1. Perform 10 repetitions of an exercise. Next, perform 10 more reps. This time, however, on the way back to the starting position, you will pause at the point of greatest contraction and tense the muscle before completing the motion. Repeat this pattern for three sets.

2. This routine is performed in the same manner as number 1. However, this version requires you to pause and tense the muscle on the way up from the starting position, rather than on the way back. Repeat this pattern for three sets.

3. Perform the movement of an exercise with dead stops (bringing the weight to a complete stop and releasing the tension in the muscle at the end of each movement) for 10 repetitions. Next, perform 10 more reps of the movement. However, on the return, pause to hold the resistance while the muscle is in its greatest state of contraction. Finally, perform another 10 reps of the exercise, pumping them out as quickly as possible. Repeat this pattern for three sets.

4. This routine is performed in the same manner as number 3. However, this version requires you to pause and tense the muscle on the way up from the starting position, rather than on the way back. Repeat this pattern for three sets.

5. For this routine, perform half the movement of an exercise (half rep) and return, followed by one full movement of the exercise (full rep). This combination is considered one complete rep. Repeat for 8 repetitions. Follow with 8 repetitions of dead stops (bringing the weight to a complete stop and releasing the tension in the muscle at the end of the movement). Next, quickly pump the resistance for 8 more repetitions.

6. Perform this routine by completing 4 full reps followed by 4 half reps. Next perform 3 full reps followed by 3 half reps. Follow this with 2 full reps, then 2 half reps. Finish with 1 full rep followed by 1 half rep.

7. For this routine, you will perform routine 6 (4 halves and 4 fulls, down to 1 half and 1 full). You will then reverse the process, starting with 1 half and 1 full progressing up to 4 halves and 4 fulls.

8. For this routine, perform 1 dead stop, followed by 1 full movement to complete one repetition. Do this for 8 reps, then 6 reps, and finish with 4 reps.

Disagreement Training (10)

Choose a weight you can do 30 full reps with. Immediately increase the weight and do 25 reps. Increase the weight and do 15 reps. Increase the weight and do 10 reps. Increase the weight and do 5 reps. Increase the weight and do 3 reps. Increase the weight and do 1 rep. Now, reverse the pattern and decrease the weight as you increase the number of reps back up to 30. Repeat the entire cycle to muscle failure.

If you are doing more than three cycles, you started with too little resistance.

Heavy/Light Training (10)

This training technique utilizes the use of alternating weights in order to work both types of muscle fiber. An example would be to complete 6 squats with 200 pounds, then go straight into 25 squats with 100 pounds. Continue this back-and-forth cycle for up to five sets.

Plyometric Suicide Sets (10)

Pick a resistance you can do 10 reps with. Complete 10 reps followed by 10 plyometric reps as described below. Rest, then repeat for a total of three sets.

The term *plyometrics* is used to describe a type of training that seeks to enhance the explosive reaction of an individual muscle contraction. The plyometric reps should be done as follows. For this example, we will use curls. Perform a complete curl, then on the way down, let the weight fall freely (do *not* let go of the weight). Halfway down, stop the weight and continue to slowly bring the bar to the starting position. This completes 1 rep.

Death by Death Training (Off the Charts)

This is *not* for the lighthearted. *Do not* attempt this routine unless you are in excellent physical condition. The goal here is simple—*to survive*. The results are astounding—some have gained a half to one full inch on their legs after only one workout. At least one training partner is required to load the plates and maintain a fast pace, without rest periods.

Using a machine, such as the incline leg press, complete 25 repetitions with as much weight as you can handle. (After some experimentation, you will be able to determine the appropriate amount of weight for each set of repetitions). While maintaining tension on the leg muscle, have your training partner add a plate to each side of the leg press. Do 15 reps. Maintain leg tension and add weight for 12 more reps. Continue to maintain tension while adding weight, and do 8 reps. Continue this pattern for 6 reps and then finally for 4 reps.

Now, get up and run as fast as you can for 125 yards, holding a barbell across the back of your shoulders. Be sure to take long strides. Stop and do 25 squats with the barbell. Hop on a leg extension machine and repeat the sequence used for the incline leg press again (25-15-12-8-6-4), adding weight after each set of repetitions.

Get up and run with the barbell, again taking long strides, for 75 yards. Stop and do 15 standing squats with the barbell. Hop on a hack-squat machine and repeat the pattern of the incline leg press, adding weight after each set.

Get up and sprint again with the barbell, this time *backward* for 50 yards. Finish with 10 standing squats.

Additional Atomic Intensity/Insanity Metabolism-Enhancing Routines

The following routines are great for burn-ing fat. They are arranged by degree of difficulty.

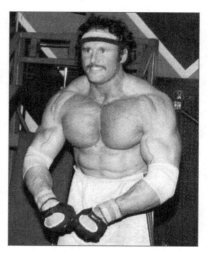

25 Reps

Pick any exercise and repeat the move-ment for 25 repetitions as fast as you can without stopping. This routine is com-plete when you can do an entire full-body workout four complete times through without adding or subtracting weight on each movement 25 times.

50 Reps

Pick any exercise and repeat the movement for 50 repetitions as fast as you can without stopping. This routine is complete when you can do an entire full body workout two complete times through without adding or subtract-ing weight on each movement 50 times.

100 Reps

Pick any exercise and repeat the movement for 100 repetitions as fast as you can without stopping. This routine is complete when you can do an entire full body workout two complete times through without adding or subtracting weight on each movement 100 times.

Super Power/Mass Building Program

Power/mass building routines combine cleans with other exercises for total-body conditioning. Cleans are performed by lifting dumbbells or barbells from the floor to your shoulders. They combine well with the overhead press, bent-over rows, and upright rows for excellent total-body conditioning in one exercise, and may be performed in the following ways:

• Straight sets of cleans (1 set, up to 25 reps)
• Cleans to overhead press (1 set, up to 25 reps)
• Cleans to bent-over row (1 set, up to 25 reps)
• Upright row to cleans (1 set, up to 25 reps)
• Cleans to front squat (1 set, up to 25 reps)

Power/mass building routines can also be performed progressively in the following ways:

• 1 clean to 1 overhead press, 2 cleans to 1 overhead press, 3 cleans to 1 overhead press, and so on, to 15 cleans
• 1 clean to 1 bent-over row, 2 cleans to 1 bent-over row, 3 cleans to 1 bent-over row, and so on, to 15 cleans
• 1 upright row to 1 clean, 2 upright rows to 1 clean, 3 upright rows to 1 clean, and so on, to 15 upright rows
• 1 clean to 1 front squat, 2 cleans to 1 front squat, 3 cleans to 1 front squat, and so on, to 15 cleans.

Super double progressive power/mass building exercises include:

• 1 clean to 1 overhead press, 2 cleans to 2 overhead presses, 3 cleans to 3 overhead presses, and so on, to 15.
• 1 clean to 1 bent-over row, 2 cleans to 2 bent-over rows, 3 cleans to 3 bent-over rows, and so on, to 15.
• 1 upright row to 1 clean, 2 upright rows to 2 cleans, 3 upright rows to 3 cleans, and so on, to 15.

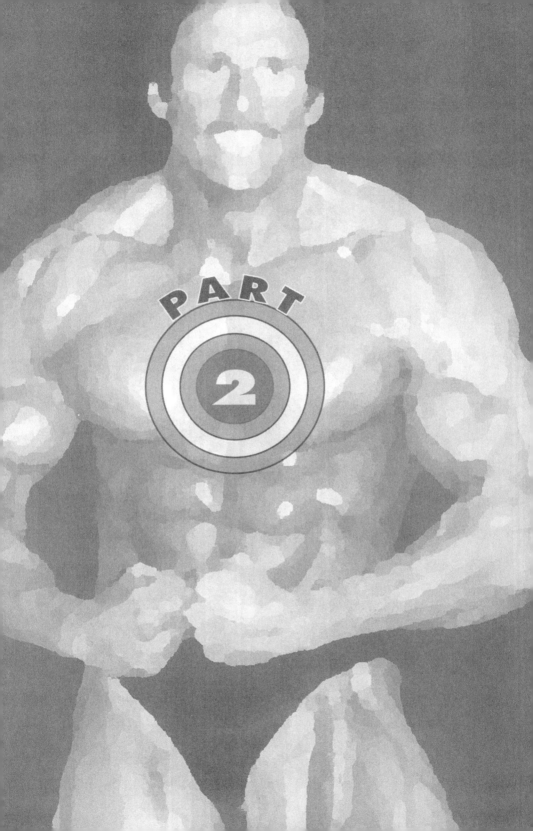

PART

2

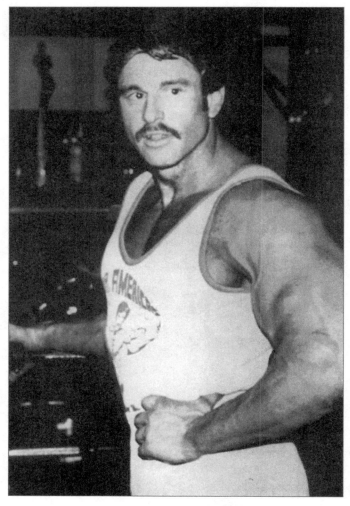

There are people who LIFT WEIGHTS . . .
and then there are those who WEIGHT LIFT!

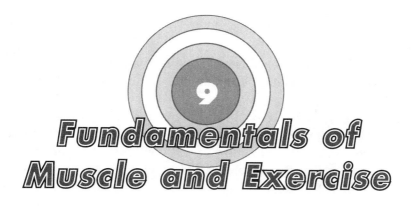

Fundamentals of Muscle and Exercise

Far from advancing, the field of exercise has been falling behind most other technologies even though there are more exercise devices and dubious inventions than ever. The very people who claim to be advancing exercise, bodybuilding, and fitness have all but destroyed them. Some celebrities and athletes who have obtained some notoriety tend to become instant experts on practically everything, but just because a celebrity is endorsing a product in a TV commercial doesn't mean the product is valid. I know, I've been there. These devices and routines, and the people selling them, are more often than not an insult to your intelligence. It is a mistake to listen to people who seldom, if ever, really understand the actual cause-and-effect relationship responsible for muscular development or weight loss.

Doubly unfortunate is that most of the published information is not based on scientifically demonstrated data. Exercise is a science. It is a study of how the body responds to a particular goal or task. What are those goals? Quite simply, they are to build a better body, a better machine—to have that machine work in an explosive manner with agility, balance, endurance, flexibility, stamina, and strength. My fitness goals are to bring harmony to the body and quiet the noise in your head so you can handle stress, both known and unknown. In doing so, you will improve your ability to increase muscle tone, lower body fat, prevent injury, ward off disease, and use your body to its fullest potential so you can tap into your reservoir of untouched power and use it beyond your wildest dreams.

In a nutshell, the goal of Atomic Fitness is to command an arsenal of physiological, psychological, and philosophical tools that, up to this point, have been lost to you. These are tools that will allow you to carry out tasks fatigue-free, with vigor and a very high level of efficiency. It is not only necessary to learn about exercise and exercise routines, but also to have a basic working knowledge of how the muscles function and how this all relates to you.

Knowledge is power. Power is a command of energy. Energy runs the universe. The more you know and realize, the more awake you become. The more awake you become, the more aware you'll be. The more aware you are, the more you can observe and the better you can act. Each bit of information obtained by you, in this case regarding exercise and muscle, is stored in the body and the mind, and will change you forever in ways seldom understood. Every cell in the body, particularly every muscle cell, is a little mind center that retains data and attempts to put that data to use, in this case, through exercise. You can never know too much, and too much is never enough.

With this in mind, it is important to understand the difference between people who lift weights and those who weight lift. Basically, it is an issue of cause and effect. People who lift weights rely on the exercise apparatus for the result. This makes them the effect, and they are causing little in the way of change. On the other hand, those who weight lift rely on the muscular contractions of the body to move a given resistance, thus causing a more positive and targeted result to the muscle. People who weight lift are causatively exercising. In lay terms, this means they are utilizing their own power to direct mental concentration into each movement, and this is far superior to relying on a machine to produce results. Achieving this higher state of awareness leads to control. Initially, when beginning to exercise, you will quickly learn you have little or no control over the contraction of the muscle groups. However, with some practice, and a good deal of awareness, you will be able to isolate the muscle groups and gain total control over them.

To be the effect of anything, whether it is exercise or situations in life, means that some outside influence is causing the result and not you. This is a *lack* of control. Being causative, however, means you are utilizing your energies and skills to create a result. You are doing the exercise. Weights or machines are only tools to increase the intensity and resistance. You should never rely on the apparatus to do the exercise; *you* do the exercise with the apparatus. In my carefully considered opinion, most currently accepted methods of exercise will never actually produce anything in the way of lasting results because they are poorly conceived. The current state of affairs encompassing the field of exercise, fitness, and conditioning is pitiful. For most individuals, the possible benefits of what is currently promoted as exercise are simply not worth the time and effort.

Exercise must be intense. You cannot increase your overall physical power by merely repeating what is already easy. You must make, with consistency, an attempt at the momentarily impossible in all exercises. This means you must exercise until it is impossible to move the resistance. Below a certain level of intensity or effort, no amount of exercise will produce enough stimulation to create positive change. On the other hand, no one should train to the point that the body cannot recover. This is where the time factor comes into play. You must train hard, but within a definite time period. It is really very simple—work as hard as possible for as brief a period as possible.

All exercise should be performed at varying speeds. At the beginning of every repetition of an exercise, you should move slowly. As the set progresses, you should try to speed up the movement, never jerking the resistance on the way up or down. Rather, move the resistance in a steady and constant motion. For example, a number of reps, let's say 8, should be selected. This doesn't mean if you can do more you shouldn't. It means complete as many as possible, in good form, and then a couple in not-so-good form. Stop only when additional movements become impossible. If the number of reps performed in good form is less than the chosen number, then use the same amount of resistance in the next workout. However, if you can perform 8 reps in good form, then the resistance should be increased for the next workout. If you continually strive to increase resistance and decrease exercise time, you'll find yourself capable of some amazing results, most notably more explosive power, endurance, and muscle mass. Such training is intensity training.

This required intensity is the basic principle in any form of worthwhile physical training. Its incredible effectiveness has been demonstrated time and again. It is perfectly clear that it works, and it is equally clear that no other currently existing style of training is capable of producing such astonishing results so quickly. For years, we have speculated that this type of training affects the survival of the muscle cells themselves because, when pushed to their maximum, they change in fear of perishing.

If you are not willing to perform highly intense exercises, you will never produce the results you could have achieved. Let's face it, nothing on this earth worth fighting for is easy. That is why there are so few real leaders and true champions. Are you one of them?

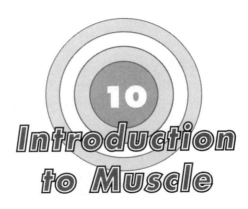

Introduction to Muscle

There are over 600 different muscles in the human body, accounting for between 40 and 50 percent of body weight. Understanding how these organs work is key to achieving optimal physical fitness. Here's why. Muscles have four distinctive traits, which collectively constitute *muscular power:* they can produce force, store energy (muscular endurance), shorten (contract) muscles at varying rates, and make muscles elastic so they will both stretch and recoil. Also important is *organic power*, which is a measure of the body's ability to supply the muscles with energy. A steady supply of energy is vital for muscles to function efficiently. Blood pumping through the body carries this energy via the digestive system to the muscles. When your muscular and organic power are developed to be as efficient as possible, you are considered physically fit.

There are many factors, including heredity and your health, that help determine your individual potential for fitness, but mental persistence is vital to improving physical capacity. Most people, for

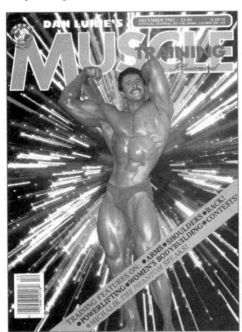

There are over 600 different muscles in the body . . . I think I found most of them.

example, could train for a lifetime and never come close to winning Mr. America simply because they lack mental persistence. They can't really believe they could do it. Personal beliefs go a long way toward producing or limiting physical change. With the Atomic Fitness System, you will discover what every great achiever knows—*concentration* is the key to success. It is critical to be absolutely single-minded, concentrating 100 percent on the muscle being exercised. You must decide what you want to accomplish and remain driven until that goal is achieved. And don't think you're too old to start exercising. That's a myth. You're never too old to begin and follow a regular exercise program. Muscle knows no age. You can rekindle that muscle tone to look and feel better. Atomic Fitness is for everyone.

You increase your physical capacity by nourishing the mind and exercising the muscles. The more you do, the more you become. By working the muscles, you boost stamina and fuel your body with energy. You increase your muscular and organic power. Regular, vigorous exercise is essential to physical and mental well-being. Unless muscles are adequately exercised or used, they will become weak and inefficient. Here are some situations that illustrate this:

■ It has been shown that a person who trains intensely is less susceptible to injuries, and if injured, recovers more rapidly.

■ It is believed that, in many cases, lower back pain is associated with weak back muscles. This is not true. It has been estimated that 90 percent of backaches can be eliminated by increasing the strength of the abdominals and the butt because, for one thing, the back muscles are supported by the abdominals. A bulging, sagging abdomen, resulting from weakened abdominal muscles, is detrimental to good posture and more often than not leads to back trauma. An unsupported back left helpless by weak gluteal muscles is trouble waiting to happen.

■ In addition to alleviating aches and pains, rigorous exercise has been shown to improve the capacity and efficiency of your heart, lungs, and other organs. The vital internal organs will actually get in shape to handle the load of an exercise regimen.

■ It has been demonstrated that intense exercise will reduce emotional and nervous tension by increasing endorphins and serotonin in the brain. This is absolutely necessary to the production of muscle.

The intensity of Atomic Fitness affects other factors for successfully building muscle, such as the development of more capillaries and nerve pathways for better and stronger nerve impulses to the muscles. This allows for greater muscle response to exercise, and maximum flushing of the muscles with blood for greater circulation, thus providing greater control over the body and its movements.

To get maximum benefits from your workouts, you must first know the workings of every muscle, how and where the muscle is attached to bone, and what exercises involve the various parts of each muscle. Every muscle has a low, middle, and high area. The slow-growing areas call for maximum concentration, while the faster-growing areas require considerably less. These areas vary according to the individual. Do not have your confidence destroyed by frustration with areas that do not have a natural tendency to build. With persistence, they will.

It is my contention, after many years of bodybuilding and observation, that mental attitude is the main ingredient to any successful endeavor. This includes building large muscles of the body. Bodybuilding and physique development are not the products of continually changing your mind. They are the result of finding the truth and sticking to it. I have found there is really only one effective way to exercise, and that is with intensity and more intensity. Concentration is key. Training without interruption allows maximum concentration and full attention to be focused on your workout—any interruption can ruin a workout by dissipating your energy. See yourself as you wish to be. If you do this, you cannot help but reach your desired goal.

WHAT IS MUSCLE AND HOW DOES IT WORK?

Muscle performs physiological activities. It has a relationship to all the other tissue cells of the body. Muscle contraction aids in supplying the numerous cells of the body with a continuous source of rebuilding materials, as well as constantly removing waste from the body. The muscles also have the unique job of supplying fluid to the tissues.

Chemical Composition of Muscle

Muscular fibers are 75 percent water, about 20 percent protein, 2 percent fat, 1 percent carbohydrates and nitrogenous extracts, and 2 percent salts, mainly potassium phosphate and carbonate.

The main virtue of exercise lies in the increase of muscular strength and tone, and the loss of body fat, as well as maintaining the normal activities of the tissues. When a muscle moves, it uses the sugar (glycogen) that is present in the muscles. During exercise, lactic acid, a waste product, accumulates and may cause a feeling of soreness or pain.

If carbonic acid and lactic acid accumulate, the muscles become acidic. If this acid accumulates in considerable amounts, the movement of the muscles will stop and so will your gains. Oxygen is required to aid continuous movement of the muscles. When oxygen comes in, the lactic acid disappears, the glycogen, or sugar, accumulates again, and the muscles become alkaline instead of acidic and continue to contract. Large amounts of oxygen are necessary for continuous work by the muscles. Eating large amounts of greens helps keep the blood alkaline and working to ward off fatigue. Developing a great aerobic capacity will allow your lungs to deliver vast amounts of oxygen to the muscle.

Anyone who is doing hard muscular work requires ten times more oxygen than when they are resting. The extra oxygen, which is provided by speeding up the circulation, increases the rate of breathing to stay ahead of oxygen debt.

During exercise, the pulse rate increases and more blood goes through the tissues. The level of increase depends on the intensity of exercise on the muscles being used. Vast amounts of blood flow, or pump, are required for the building of muscle and the burning of fat.

The ability to reduce length upon stimulation is most highly developed in muscle tissue. This property, together with elasticity, enables these tissues

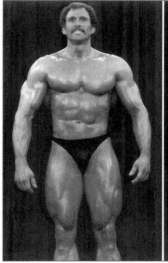
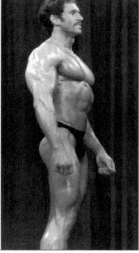

In order to build muscle, a sufficient amount of oxygen is paramount.

to shorten (contract) and then return to their original length (relax). Muscle tissue is responsible for all movement in the body.

There are three kinds of muscle tissue: skeletal, smooth, and cardiac. Although all three types have features in common, each has additional characteristics that suit it for its special work in the body.

Size and Shape

Muscles vary in size, shape, and arrangement of fibers. Those that allow considerable range of movement are long and narrow, whereas those requiring strength of movement over a shorter range are short and broad. In their simplest arrangement, muscles are composed of a bundle of parallel fibers, usually tapered at both ends.

Attachments

As in the case of facial muscles that control expression, muscles are generally attached to other muscles, or to skin, by connective tissue. Many other muscles are attached to the bones. They move by a narrow strip of dense connective tissue called aponeurosis. Still, others, such as those found in the voice box of the throat, attach to cartilage.

It is important to remember that a muscle can produce movement only by *pulling* on a body part, never by pushing. The end of a muscle that remains stationary during the pulling action is called the origin. The opposite end, where the movement of the body part takes place, is the insertion. Although muscles can only pull, some muscles can move either of their two ends, thus reversing origin and insertion designations. Muscles usually move a body part by pulling across a joint, as in bending the knee or elbow.

Generally, muscles do not act alone, but in groups that affect a particular movement. Certain muscles in the group are primarily responsible for the action. These are the prime movers. Other muscles in the group, called synergists, assist the prime movers, often by stabilizing the joint involved. When one group of muscles contracts to perform a particular action, such as flexing the elbow, the muscle group that opposes this action (the extensors of the elbow) are called the antagonists, and they must be relaxed.

This interaction of various muscles allows for the smooth, coordinated movement of body parts. In the extremities, the bulk of a muscle is not directly located over the part of the body being moved by it because, in order to achieve maximum range and leverage, most of the muscle mass will lie next to the joint over which it acts. For example, the biceps brachii, which flexes the supinated forearm, lies on the anterior surface of the arm. Also, some muscles, such as the biceps femoris, hamstrings, quadriceps, and sartorius, span two joints, the hip and the knee.

Names of Muscles

The name of a muscle often gives a clue to its action. Muscles may be named according to the number of heads of origin, for example the biceps (a two-headed muscle) and the triceps (a three-headed muscle). Muscles may also be named according to their geometric shape, such as the trapezius, which is shaped like a trapezoid. Perhaps the most informatively named muscles are those that refer to their place of attachment in the body. One such muscle is the sternocleidomastoid, which is attached to the sternum, the clavicle, and the mastoid of the temporal bone.

Chemical Changes in Muscle

Muscles are machines that convert chemical energy into mechanical energy. Part of the energy involved in muscle contraction results in movement and part is given off as heat. The movement of skeletal muscles is a very important method of heat production in the body. The efficiency factor of muscle, that is, the percentage of energy actually resulting in work or movement, is about 25 percent, and this factor compares very favorably with the efficiency of most man-made machines.

Oxygen Debt and Fatigue

In strenuous muscular exercise, the chemical steps previously described take place without the presence of oxygen, which means they are anaerobic. This occurs when, during prolonged or strenuous exercise, a person is not able to breathe in enough oxygen to satisfy the requirements of the muscles. This inability results in an oxygen debt being accumulated in the body. For example, anyone using the Atomic Fitness System requires large quantities of oxygen; yet, during the time it takes to train, the person can absorb only about one-sixth that amount.

This oxygen debt is paid back during the rest or recovery period following the exercise. While recovering, the trainee will breathe rapidly and deeply. The oxygen taken in is then used to remove the lactic acid that accumulates in the muscle during anaerobic contraction.

As lactic acid piles up and the supply of energy-producing materials becomes depleted, the ability of the muscle to contract gradually becomes depressed. This loss of ability to contract leads to a condition called fatigue, in which the muscle contractions become weaker and weaker. The oxygen taken in during the recovery period is required for the removal of lactic acid, part of which is broken down into carbon dioxide and water. Energy is released during this breakdown and is used to change the rest of the lactic acid to glycogen, thus replenishing the energy-producing compounds necessary for contraction.

In order for a muscle to get shorter and thicker, or to fully contract, it has to first have proper stimulation. In receiving this stimulation, as in lifting a weight, irritability, or the exciting of the muscle, can bring about its special function, which can consist of intensifying, stretching, and contracting the muscle. These are the major functions that make up the characteristics of muscle tissue.

Muscle Tone

Even when skeletal muscles are completely relaxed, a varying amount of firmness or tension remains. This state of continued partial contraction in all healthy muscles is called muscle tone. It is produced by the simultaneous action of different motor units scattered throughout the muscle. These motor-unit groups contract in relays. It is probably the only aspect of skeletal muscle that you cannot control voluntarily. When the nerve supply to a muscle is destroyed, or muscles are overworked, the muscle fibers will no longer react to nerve stimuli. This will cause muscle to lose its tone and become flaccid. The muscle will actually waste away.

Muscle contraction is concerned with the tone of the muscle cells, which is maintained by the chemical and physical composition of tissue fluids and by the nervous system. The brain (specifically, the cerebellum) makes the final adjustments necessary for muscle groups to act. Muscles are supplied with two types of nerve fibers—sensory fibers conveying the state of contraction to the central nervous system, and motor fibers conveying impulses from the central nervous system to the muscles, controlling their contraction.

Response to Stimuli

It has been found that if the force applied to a single muscle fiber is strong enough, it will produce a maximum contraction. This is the all-or-nothing law, and it means that each muscle fiber gives a maximal response or none at all. Although fatigue and varying conditions of nutrition can alter the cell's response, increasing the force of the stimulus will ensure the greatest response. The muscle-fiber response is called muscle recruitment. It is, of course, optimal to recruit as many muscle fibers as possible during exercise, and the Atomic Fitness System uses maximum recruitment techniques to their fullest.

When a muscle is stimulated to contract many times in succession, the contractions increase progressively at first. This effect is determined by an increase in irritability. However, as metabolic waste products increase, irritability decreases, and the contractions diminish progressively until fatigue develops. The diminishing effect occurs much more rapidly when exercise is done slowly. With the Atomic Fitness System, a lot of this metabolic shutdown is avoided.

Source of Stimulus for Contraction

In order to contract, or shorten, skeletal muscle must be stimulated. This is best accomplished by providing the greatest force possible in the shortest period of time. This stimulation is provided by motor-nerve fibers coming from the voluntary part of the central nervous system, which can be monitored by the mind. A motor-nerve fiber plus the muscle fibers is called a motor unit. One nerve fiber may supply from one to two hundred muscle fibers, depending on the type of work the muscle is called upon to perform. This is why it is absolutely necessary to apply different angles when developing your training routine.

Types of Contraction

In the body, there are two types of muscle contractions involved in fitness routines—*isotonic* and *isometric*. When a muscle becomes shorter and thicker, but its tone remains the same, the contraction is referred to as isotonic. If, however, the muscle is forced to respond against some resistance that it cannot lift or move, the contraction is referred to as isometric.

Contractions in Skeletal Muscles

Contractions of skeletal muscles are usually isotonic, but certain tasks involve the coordinated development of both isometric and isotonic contractions of a muscle. The height of contraction of a skeletal muscle is in direct proportion to the strength of the force applied. This is not a contradiction of the all-or-nothing law. It is explained by the fact that muscle cells are separate units insulated from one another by connective tissue, which react to the force brought to bear on them. Contraction and relaxation of muscles are also influenced by concentrations of potassium and salt within the cells and interstitial fluids. Magnesium and calcium are essential for a normal response of skeletal muscle fibers to the nerve impulse. A lack of calcium ions increases irritability and may affect muscle relaxation. Muscles must relax in order to recover after exercise; this is the only way muscle grows. Magnesium has a sedative action on the neuromuscular junction, which helps the skeletal muscle fibers repair. As you can see, a knowledge of nutrition is essential to understanding why muscles fail.

Conditions of Contraction

Skeletal muscle contracts quickly and relaxes promptly. It responds favorably to intense actions. The contraction of a skeletal muscle is the result of stimuli discharged by the nerve fibers. By increasing the stimuli, you increase the resulting contraction. There is a brief period after the muscle is stimulated, before it contracts, and this is called the latent period. It is followed by a period of contraction, in turn followed by a period of relaxation.

In general, the stronger the stimulus, the stronger the contraction will be. If you apply a greater level of intensity to the muscle, a greater number of single cells will contract. The strongest contractions result from moderate to fast rates of stimuli. A long duration of a repetition will result in a decreased level of contraction. Some load is necessary in order to get the best response; however, increasing the load beyond the optimum level decreases the level of contractions. Heavy weights do not build muscle.

Muscles do their best work at an optimum body temperature, about 98.6°F (37°C). If the body temperature is raised much above this, the muscle loses its excitability and becomes functionally depressed, entering a state of heat rigor. This is a condition of permanent shortening. Therefore, a training facility must be cool and ventilated, and training gear must allow the body to breathe.

Source of Energy for Muscle Contraction

Carbohydrates, stored in the muscle in a complex form called glycogen, are the source of energy for muscle contraction. When energy is needed, glycogen is broken down to the simple sugar glucose, which can be burned by the muscle to produce energy.

A trigger mechanism is needed, however, to allow the transfer of this energy to the protein molecules that make up the muscle fiber. This mechanism involves two other substances found in muscle, phosphocreatine and adenosine triphosphate (ATP). The latter is capable of storing large amounts of energy, some of which combines with calcium ions to form the trigger complex. This complex causes the muscle tissue to become irritable so it will respond to stimuli.

Fueling Muscle Contraction

ATP is the immediate source of energy for muscle contraction. Although a muscle fiber contains only enough ATP to power a few contractions, its ATP supply is constantly replenished. There are three sources of high-energy phosphate to keep the ATP supplies adequate: creatine phosphate, glycogen, and cellular respiration in the mitochondria of the fibers.

Creatine Phosphate

The phosphate group in creatine phosphate is attached by a highly energized bond similar to that of ATP. Creatine phosphate derives its high-energy phosphate from ATP and has the ability to donate it back to adenosine diphosphate (ADP) to form ATP. In short, creatine phosphate + ADP $\longleftrightarrow$ creatine + ATP. The supply of creatine phosphate in the fiber is about ten times larger than that of ATP and therefore serves as a modest reservoir of ATP.

Glycogen

Skeletal muscle fibers contain about 1 percent glycogen (sugar). The muscle fiber can break this glycogen down into fuel, which enters the energy pathway to yield a pair of ATP molecules for each pair of lactic-acid molecules. This small amount of glycogen is enough to keep the muscle functioning if it fails to receive sufficient oxygen to meet its ATP needs by respiration. This is why good overall physical conditioning is absolutely necessary for building large muscle. If you go into oxygen debt, your muscles will fail. This glycogen source is limited and eventually the muscle must depend on cellular respiration. If the body cannot supply enough oxygen to meet sugar needs, then the sugar burns off, but the lactic acid remains, leaving the body with muscle soreness.

Cellular Respiration

Cellular respiration is not only required to meet the ATP needs of a muscle involved in prolonged activity (thereby causing more rapid and deeper breathing), but is also required after exercise to enable the body to resynthesize glycogen from the lactic acid produced earlier (deep breathing continues for a time after exercise is stopped). The body must repay its oxygen debt.

Summation

If several stimuli are sent rapidly into a muscle, they will combine to produce a strong contraction. Adding individual muscle twitches together in this way is called summation and it occurs in two ways:

1. By increasing the frequency of nerve impulses coming down the nerve fiber.

2. By increasing the number of motor units responding.

Both are strongly activated by the Atomic Fitness System.

The Special Features of Skeletal Muscle

I would like to reiterate the necessity of learning all about the item you are trying to get control over, in this case skeletal muscle, which is the largest category of muscle tissue in the body. These muscle fibers show alternating light and dark bands called striations, which result from the periodic spacing of the protein molecules that comprise the fibers, and are visible when fat and water are absent in the muscle and skin. Each fiber is considered one cell, and it can vary in length from 1 to 80 millimeters. Several fibers are bound together in bundles by connective tissue. Smaller bundles are bound together into larger bundles called fascia, and these bundles constitute skeletal muscle. Because these muscles are supplied by the part of the nervous system that is under the direct control of the will, they are said to be voluntary.

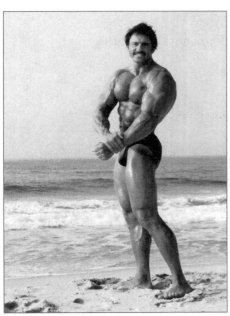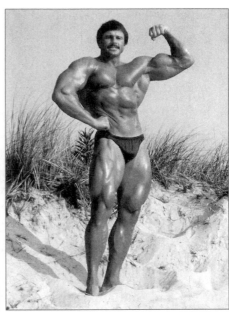

The more you do, the more you become.

Type I versus Type II Fibers

The two different types of muscle fiber found in most skeletal muscles, types I and II, differ in their structure and biochemistry.

Type I fibers, also known as *slow-twitch* fibers, are:

- activated by small-diameter motor neurons, and are therefore slow-conducting;
- dependent on cellular respiration for energy production;
- dominant in muscles that depend on tonus, for example, those responsible for posture and endurance;
- loaded with mitochondria;
- resistant to fatigue; and
- rich in myoglobin, therefore red in color.

Type II fibers, also known as *fast-twitch* fibers, are:

- activated by large diameter motor neurons, therefore fast-conducting;

- dependent on glycolysis for ATP production;
- dominant in muscles used for rapid movement and power;
- low in mitochondria;
- easily fatigued;
- low in myoglobin, therefore whitish in color; and
- rich in glycogen.

Most skeletal muscles contain a mixture of both types of fibers. However, a single motor unit always contains one or the other, never both. The ratio of type I to type II fibers in the muscle can be changed with endurance training, producing more fatigue-resistant type I fibers.

Hypertrophy

Forceful and continued muscular activity causes the muscle fibers to increase in size. This growth is called muscle hypertrophy and is the goal of exercise. In addition to an increase in fiber size, the muscle gains more of the energy-producing compounds involved in muscle contraction: ATP, glycogen, and creatine phosphate, thus increasing the body's energy. Hypertrophy is a normal response of all healthy muscle tissue to usage.

Atrophy

The opposite of muscular hypertrophy is muscular atrophy. This decrease in fiber size and the amount of nutrients present occurs when a muscle is not used for any reason. If a body part has been immobilized for a period of time, it undergoes disuse atrophy. If the motor nerve to a skeletal muscle is cut (this is known as denervation), atrophy begins immediately. Unless passive stretching is applied daily to such a muscle, the fibers tend to shorten in length, and even if the nerve supply gets reestablished, the fibers are permanently shortened and of little use.

THOUGHTS ON THE MUSCULAR SYSTEM

Muscle is a living substance, and as with all other living matter, there are some basic facts you must learn if you expect them to grow. I outline them below.

Rest and Recovery

Though probably the least thought-about factors in muscle growth, rest and recovery are, in my opinion, the most important. Maximum pump involving the same muscle(s) in every workout does not build muscle tissue. It takes seventy-two hours to rebuild muscle tissue after it's been worked because you grow only during periods of rest. So, you must be sure to rest adequately between workouts to permit muscle repair and growth. There is physical rest and mental rest, and each is equally important. When you go without physical rest, it can cause stress. Stress uses up proteins, fats, and carbohydrates, which are all ingredients of growing muscle. Mental stress is worse. It can produce a response of the hormones cortisone and adrenaline that can run you into the ground and ruin your life. When you train, you break down large amounts of body tissue that the body must replace to prepare for your next workout. This is how you grow, and rest, sleep, and tranquility are essential in the rebuilding process.

During a workout, digestion mostly stops, so it is useless to eat before a workout. The muscles during exercise are working vigorously to achieve your appointed goal, keeping food from reaching the muscle. This is why eating and allowing digestion to occur during periods of rest is necessary to replace the cellular chemicals and speed the ingredients of replenishment to you.

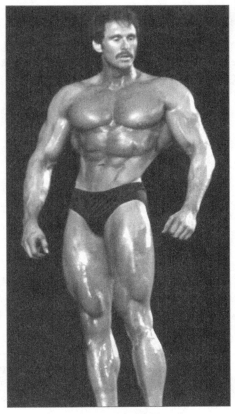

How much rest do you need? The answer is different for everyone. You have to experiment to see just what you need. In regard to sleep, about eight to ten hours a night is generally an adequate amount for most people. When you are trying to gain size, it is essential to abstain completely from physical activities on off days.

The Symmetry of Muscle

There is no reason why a fast rate of muscle growth cannot be maintained to the point of the individual's potential. Most people interested in muscle conditioning do either too little or too much exercise. They fall into a rut, never becoming aware that intensity training is better. In fact, the harder you train, the less time you need. This brings us to the second leg of the Atomic Fitness routine—recovery.

The body responds well to hard exercise, and recovers easily. It does poorly when even a poor level of exercise is done for too long a time period. Although you can't overtrain, you can work overtime. Results are achieved when the body has time for muscle growth and removal of waste. Muscle size is accomplished when the body's reserves are high. When the reserves are low or exhausted, as happens with an incorrect training routine, the system is no longer able to meet the requirements for change, and the muscular nervous system shuts down.

When you have worked the muscle to failure, with an intense, strict, little-rest style of training, the muscles and related systems need time to recover. The body makes certain demands for material required for growth. The primary limiting factor in creating the ultimate body via exercise is the ability of the body's systems to make the chemical changes within an allotted time period. If you work out too slowly, little or nothing in the way of growth and conditioning can occur.

Hard Work Induces Change— Time Allows That Change to Happen!

First, within the human system, there exist a number of regulatory subsystems whose functions aid conditioning and recovery. I have tried to bring their purposes and functions to your attention, so you would have a better-than-average working knowledge of how exercise and recovery play into your goals of obtaining the ultimate physique.

Recovery is simply a matter of supply and demand. If the supply (rest and proper nutrition) is not available to recover, the body will reduce its ability to demand (muscle growth). It is this demand, or command, that influences change. It is immensely important for you to understand that intense exertion is required to induce physical change. Low intensity (intensity being the most amount of work possible in the shortest possible time) produces low, if any, results. Smart, hard work is required. Your recovery ability is limited, so keep those workouts fast, hard, and brief, with two days between body parts to rest and recover. A failure to understand these principles has led to the present debacle in exercise circles. Trainers work their clients too much, never too hard. Intensity, under the guidelines of the routine, matters. Quick in–quick out builds a better body throughout.

Exercise is designed to induce a positive hormone balance in the body— it is the positive hormones that burn fat and build muscle, and they have a limited application time in the body. Approximately forty-five minutes after the start of exercise, the negative hormones, as I call them, start to kick in to kind of protect you from yourself. Under the negative hormone response, little muscle gain or fat burning is possible. Therefore, long, drawn-out workouts followed by overlong rest periods between sets are not just useless, they are dangerous.

Atomic Fitness intensity training is beneficial because it sharply reduces training time. It should be clearly understood, however, that intensity training is not merely an attempt to save training time, it is an absolute requirement for producing the best results possible due to the extremely short recovery-time factors encountered in muscular activity and positive hormone response. In order to work a particular muscle as hard as it must be worked to induce maximum growth stimulation, while staying within the limits imposed by the overall recovery ability of the system, you must use Atomic Fitness–type training routines. When this is done properly, only a few, brief training sessions are required, or even desirable. Doing more will not induce more growth stimulation.

Second, nutrition is more or less 80 percent of all your rebuilding efforts. Rebuilding depends on your metabolism (the rate at which your body functions) after you have trained and are resting. In order for your muscles to gain size and strength, they need good nutrition to enter the bloodstream as fast as possible, and to achieve this, a balance of food and supplements are necessary. Proteins build muscle; carbohydrates provide energy for training; fats, vitamins, and minerals are necessary for digestion. When to eat and how to eat are also important. In order to achieve your goal, it is vital to know the right amounts and combinations of foods to eat. (*See* Chapters 13–17.)

Third, muscle shape is the greatest factor in your body's appearance. Your basic muscular insertions and origins determine how you look and how strong you are. It should be noted that, although structural considerations make it nearly impossible to change the shape of a muscle, the illusion of change can be accomplished. I've seen it and I've done it. For example, a long, thick bicep can be changed into a high-peaked bicep by performing curls in a certain manner to develop the tie-in from the front deltoid to the upper bicep. Another example is the pectoralis muscles. Due to structural difficulties, a high, wide, and square pectoralis cannot be changed to a round, thick pectoralis. However, surrounding muscles can be modified, thereby creating the desired illusion. The reverse is also true. All the wide chest work in the world is not going to give you that wide sweep in your chest. The illusion of this can be created, however, by not overdeveloping the neck, trapezius, and oblique areas. You should develop a large rib cage, upper back, and upper thigh area—this will help give you an hourglass appearance.

Another problem area is usually the calves. These areas can be developed, but unfortunately, they will never look as good as naturally developed lower legs. You can, however, create an illusion to make the calf look fuller. The inner calf is the beauty of the lower leg. To compensate for high

The Properties of Muscle

■ Muscle accomplishes movement by its ability to lengthen and shorten, by its ability to recruit fiber to complete a task. The greater the demand or intensity, the greater the level of muscle-fiber recruitment.

■ This recruitment produces movement by exerting force on tendons, which pulls on bones.

■ All muscles pull via a joint.

■ Strength is the coordinated effort of that muscle pulling, working together with other muscles.

■ The more muscle fibers, the stronger the pulling force.

■ Muscle pulls from its origin, where it starts, to its insertion, where it finishes.

■ All muscles have opposing muscles. Movers and opposers work together to create control.

■ Balance (synergy) between the mover and the opposer create the greatest effect of movement.

■ If you contract the opposer, you will recruit more mover.

or small inner calves, you can develop the outer calf regions and frontal calf areas. You'll be surprised at how much you can do to change the appearance of your calves.

Finally, posture is important. Always try to be conscious of how you sit and stand. Good posture helps you maintain your overall health as well as adequate nerve and blood flow to and from your brain. To maintain upright posture, human skeletal muscles are always in a state of partial contraction. If the muscles begin to relax and stretch, an unconscious reflex takes place to keep your balance and your posture.

Specialized muscle fibers contain sensory spiral nerves, and when stimulated by the muscle stretch, they send impulses to the spinal cord. Motor nerves are then activated, and impulses travel back to the muscle fibers, causing them to contract. Through this rapid *stretch reflex*, the balance between opposing muscle groups is maintained. Since many muscles may

■ Muscle tone equals the degree of constant tension on the muscle between movers and opposers, which leads to constant muscle readiness, which equals explosive power, enduring stamina, strength, and size.

■ This leads to speed over a range of motion, which equals force.

■ Force equals torque.

■ Torque equals power.

■ Power monitors control.

■ Control monitors ability.

■ Ability is the precursor to skill.

■ Skill in exercise produces the optimum effects.

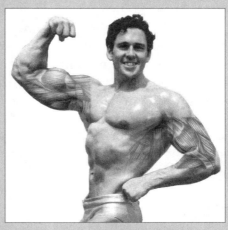

■ The goal is to get the muscle to do as much work as possible in the shortest period of time.

Please read this inset as many times as necessary to fully understand the nature and motion of muscle—time, space, energy.

be involved in any postural change, sensory impulses are sent to the lower brain to coordinate the stretch reflex.

Why is Atomic Fitness necessary? Because it is impossible to realize your full potential without a planned program of exercise. Your muscles are required to deliver force, speed, and accuracy time after time. This requires physical fitness, which means that the body needs to be at the highest level of conditioning. Anything below this standard will become the weak link in your success because it can only encourage poor health, aches and pains, lots of stress, and premature aging.

For optimal play, a properly planned program of exercise is essential. Regardless of your age or sex, a well-planned Atomic Fitness program provides the fastest and the most effective way to improve your body and your health. Trained muscles are stronger, faster, and more explosive. Intense exercise will increase muscle reaction time as well as prevent injury. Intense exercise has been proven to decrease anxiety and improve your concentration.

In my opinion, no other function can affect the internal organs of the body more profoundly than the Atomic Fitness System. Using this system can strengthen health, improve circulation and the digestive system, provide optimum lung power, and strengthen bone. In order to perform the Atomic Fitness System of training, you must have optimum conditioning.

Atomic Fitness training will strengthen and align your structure, assuring proper posture, thereby allowing muscle to attain maximum symmetry. Posture is one of the most important considerations of Atomic conditioning. It is, after all, your frame and structure on which all else depends. A sound structure provides the body with the necessary balance it needs to perform tasks easily. Your entire body works under the principles of balance. Poor muscle tone is the main ingredient of a collapsing structure, leading to poor posture and loss of bone tissue. A weak structure leads to arthritis and can shorten your life. It is important for anyone who wishes to gain as many years as possible not to overlook this program, which I've designed to ensure structural balance.

11

Basic Anatomy & Physiology and the Training Effect

I t is not necessary to know how a car works in order to drive it, but the body is much more than just a machine you occupy, and a basic knowledge of it will give you a profound understanding of what you're living in. The human body is a biomechanical machine, and if you want to build a better machine, you had better understand what's at stake. This machine requires maintenance and upgrading. Unfortunately, although it is critical to understand how the body responds to training and conditioning, as well as the role each part plays in this quest, the human body does not come with a maintenance manual. So how do you keep it performing at maximum efficiency when you know little about its main components?

The brief, to-the-point information in this chapter will provide valuable insights into the components involved in maintaining your body's condition and fitness levels. Knowledge is power. Harness this power and you will reap the benefits.

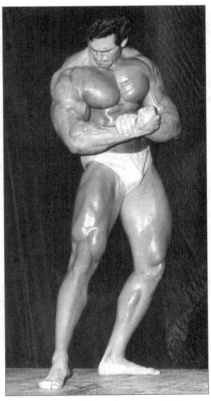

Knowledge is power.

CELLS AND TISSUE

Cells are the basic structural and functional units of an organism. There are
many types of cells in the body, each differentiated by its assigned role. Each
cell is like a small factory with receiving and shipping storerooms and
power plants. These factories require nutrition and oxygen to run.

The next level of structure in the body is tissue. This is made up of
groups of cells that perform special functions. Exercise fires up the cells, and
groups of cells (tissue), keeping them rich with blood, nutrients, and oxygen. Exercise keeps cells and tissues in a healthy state. If you don't exercise
your body, it will deteriorate, starting at the cellular level. Premature aging
of bones and muscles is a direct result of cellular inactivity and is brought
about by poor circulation of blood, nutrition, and oxygen. Exercise stimulates, refreshes, and rejuvenates these tissues.

BLOOD

The bloodstream is the body's assembly line. Red blood cells are the carriers
for all the blood, filling up and then emptying their contents to return again
for a refill. Hemoglobin carries the oxygen in the red blood cells, and the
number of available cells determines the body's vitality. Exercise increases
this number, resulting in more hemoglobin, which in turn produces more
oxygen and more vitality. It stands to reason that a well-conditioned body
will have a greater volume of blood to work with, thereby enriching all the
cells and removing their waste products.

Exercise is responsible for the development of new vascular passage-
ways, which aid in endurance and fatigue fighting. Exercise increases the
size of the blood vessels, allowing for unrestricted flow and helping in the
control of blood pressure.

ORGANS

Different types of tissues are joined together to form organs. There are many
different organs of structure and function. The only organs you need to concern yourself with are those that will aid in your conceptual understanding
of exercise conditioning and emotion.

Organs of Digestion

The organs of digestion include the stomach, the intestines, the pancreas,
the liver, and the kidneys.

Stomach

The stomach is a J-shaped enlargement of the gastrointestinal tract, located directly under the diaphragm in the left region of the abdomen. The inlet is the throat. The outlet is the intestines. When empty, it is about the size of a sausage; when filled with food, however, it can stretch to an incredible size. The passage of solid or semisolid food from mouth to stomach takes approximately four to eight seconds. Soft foods and liquids take only a second.

The stomach mixes the food into a sort of pulp, using a wave motion. The primary chemical activity of the stomach is to begin the digestion of protein through the use of the enzyme pepsin, which can only operate in an acidic environment—it becomes inactive in an alkaline environment. Protein promotes an acidic environment. Starch and carbohydrates promote an alkaline environment.

Note: Fats rely almost exclusively on enzymes found in the small intestine.

The stomach empties all its contents two to six hours after ingestion. Foods rich in carbohydrates leave the stomach in a few hours. Proteins are somewhat slower. The process is slowest after fats have been consumed. An athlete will perform at his or her best on an empty stomach after all digestion is completed and the blood has delivered the nutrients to their respective destinations. Muscles rich with blood, oxygen, and nutrients will perform at their absolute peak. Food that is undigested or going through the digestive process will rob the muscle cells of their vitality because the blood is being used in the digestive tract. Since the digestive process requires a great amount of energy from start to finish, exercising while it is taking place cannot serve you very well.

Intestines

Although the stomach does participate in the absorption of alcohol, electrolytes, some drugs, and water, most food absorption takes place in the intestines. The small intestine is where most chemical digestion takes place, aided by the gallbladder, liver, and pancreas.

Pancreas

The pancreas is a gland made up of clusters of cells. It is linked to the small intestines by a series of ducts. One percent of these cells form the endocrine portion of the pancreas, secreting the hormones glucagon, insulin, and somatostatin. The remaining 99 percent of cells release a mixture of digestive enzymes designed to digest specific foods.

Liver

The next organ in line is the liver. It is located under the diaphragm and occupies most of the right portion of the abdomen. It is divided into right and left lobes that are separated by a ligament. The liver, like the pancreas, is connected to the small intestine by a series of ducts. The lobes of the liver are made up of functional units. These units destroy worn-out white and red blood cells and bacteria. Oxygen, most nutrients, and certain poisons are extracted by liver cells. Nutrients are stored or used to make new materials. Poisons are stored or detoxified. Products made by the liver and nutrients needed by other cells are secreted back into the blood.

The liver performs many vital functions.

- It manufactures bile salts, which are used in the small intestine for the emulsification and absorption of fats. It is impossible to lose body fat if the liver is overworked or not functioning to its capacity.

- Along with mast cells, it manufactures most of the other plasma proteins.

- It destroys worn-out red and white blood cells and some bacteria.

- Its cells contain enzymes that either break poisons down or transform them into less harmful compounds. When amino acids are burned for energy, for example, they leave behind toxic nitrogenous wastes, such as ammonia, that are converted to urea by the liver cells. Moderate amounts of urea are harmless to the body and are easily excreted by the kidneys and sweat glands.

- It collects newly absorbed nutrients. Depending on the body's needs, it can change any excess monosaccharides into glycogen or fat, both of which can be stored. Or it can transform glycogen, fat, and protein into glucose.

- It stores copper, glycogen, iron, and vitamins A, D, E, and K. It also stores some poisons that cannot be broken down and excreted. (High levels of DDT are found in the livers of animals, including humans, who eat sprayed fruits and vegetables.)

- Along with the kidneys, it participates in the activation of vitamin D.

In short, the liver is what builds muscle. All the training in the world will do you no good if the liver is not up to the task.

Kidneys

The paired kidneys are reddish organs that resemble kidney beans in shape. They are found just above the waist near the posterior wall of the abdomen.

The metabolism of nutrients results in the production of wastes by body cells, including carbon dioxide and excess water and heat. Protein catabolism (the breaking down of molecules for energy) produces toxic nitrogenous wastes, such as ammonia and urea. In addition, many of the essential ions, such as chloride, hydrogen, phosphate, sodium, and sulfate, tend to accumulate in excess of the body's needs. All the toxic materials and the excess essential materials must be eliminated.

The primary function of the urinary system, and thereby the kidneys, is to help keep the body in homeostasis by controlling the composition and volume of the blood. It does so by removing and restoring selected amounts of water and solutes (dissolved substances). As the kidneys go about their activities, they remove many materials from the blood, return the ones the body requires, and eliminate the rest. The eliminated materials are collectively called urine. The entire volume of blood in the body is filtered by the kidneys approximately sixty times a day.

Heart

The heart is the center of the cardiovascular system. It is a hollow, muscular organ that weighs about 11 ounces and beats over 100,000 times a day to pump blood through the equivalent of more than 60,000 miles of blood vessels. The blood vessels form a network of tubes that carry blood from the heart to the tissues of the body and then return it to the heart.

The heart is situated obliquely between the lungs. It is shaped like a blunt cone about the size of your closed fist. This is the magnificent engine that keeps the whole assembly line going. It takes oxygen-laden blood from the lungs and pumps it throughout the body, while at the same time taking carbon dioxide–laden blood back from the body and pumping it into the lungs where it is exchanged for more oxygen.

The heart began its work before you were born. It is working now, and will continue to work your entire life. Ironically, when you give it little to do, the heart works less efficiently than it does when you make it work more. An unconditioned heart beats harder and less efficiently than a conditioned heart performing the same activity. Obesity, stress, and many other factors can increase your heart rate considerably, even though you may appear to be in great condition. Even at complete rest, an unconditioned person who does not exercise forces his or her heart to beat an extra 30,000 times daily.

The heart tissue is all muscle. Unlike the lungs, the heart does its own work—unquestionably the most important work in the body. The health of its tissue depends on its size and how well it is supplied with blood vessels. An athlete's heart is generally strong and healthy. It is relatively large and highly efficient, pumping more blood with less effort. Like any top athlete, it accomplishes great things with seemingly effortless ease. A conditioned heart is beautifully resilient and, if you could see it, would be a beautiful thing to watch.

A healthy heart is characterized, first, by a conspicuously favorable blood supply provided by large, healthy, blood-supply routes. For its own energy requirements, the heart needs the same supply of oxygen that it pumps to the other tissues in the body. Healthy cardiac tissue depends on saturation from large blood-supply routes. This saturation, or vascularization, is one of the most important benefits of the training effect, and nowhere is this more evident, or more important, than in the heart.

The next factor that indicates the health of the heart is the heart rate. As they grow larger and stronger, conditioned hearts can beat more slowly because they're pumping more blood with each stroke. Exercise reduces maximum heart rates, which is important. Healthy hearts will peak, without strain, at 190 beats per minute or less, while poorly conditioned hearts may go as high as 220 beats or more during exhausting activity. This is dangerously high. Exercise can strengthen the heart so it can hold near-maximum rates for longer periods before fatigue sets in.

One of the factors affecting heart rate is the anticipatory, or tension, rate. You might think of it as the emotional heart rate. It is this ability to respond to mental, as well as physical, stimuli that makes the heart such a unique muscle. Crisis does affect the heart rate, but training can reduce this effect.

Two systems in your body prepare you for the "fight or flight" response by starting the heart pumping to rush in more oxygen before you've even made a move. In periods of acute emotional stress, the nervous system speeds up most of the body's activities and combines with the adrenal glands to provide a high level of hormones for the blood. When these hormones reach the heart, they cause it to increase in rate and strength of contraction.

A deconditioned heart does not always have the ability to slow down after a sudden stimulus. The heart may continue to beat at an excessively fast rate that could possibly lead to a heart attack. With a conditioned heart, there's a better balance. You can encounter a sudden stimulus and still maintain control—a high, potentially damaging level of hormones is simply never reached.

This, too, is part of the training effect. Either due to decreased production or to a more efficient utilization of hormones, a conditioned body is less affected by them. Add to this the fact that a conditioned heart is already trained to level off at a relatively low maximum rate, and you have built-in protection against an uncontrollable emotional crisis. A deconditioned body doesn't have this protection. If a person also tends to be hyperreactive (someone who gets overexcited, even in minor emergencies), then that person has two problems—too much emotion and too little built-in physical protection.

The training effect benefits the heart in several ways by developing a strong, healthy muscle that works more effortlessly during moments of crisis or times of peak physical exertion. By doing so, the heart maintains large reserves of power to handle whatever physical or emotional stress is imposed on it.

Lungs

Air consists of 21 percent oxygen and 79 percent nitrogen, and the amount you can process (bring in and push out) is the first limiting factor in exercise. Lungs have no muscles of their own. They depend completely on the diaphragm and rib cage muscles, and the stronger these muscles, the greater the lung's capacity to consume oxygen.

The amount of air you can exhale after a deep breath is known as the lung's vital capacity. A conditioned body will utilize much more of its lung capacity than one in poor condition.

The air that remains consistently in your lungs is referred to as residual volume. It is difficult to exhale too much of the residual volume; therefore, this will limit the amount of air you can breathe in, causing shortness of breath. If there is a large volume of residual air in the lungs, it will prevent that portion of the lungs from working properly. The usable portion of your lungs will be limited if you allow your body to deteriorate by being out of shape. No matter how nutritionally sound you are, you can only perform physically up to the capacity of your lungs.

SLEEP

Humans need sleep. They sleep and awaken in a fairly constant twenty-four-hour cycle. Just as there are different levels of consciousness, there are different levels of sleep. Normal sleep consists of two levels, non-rapid eye movement (non-REM) and rapid eye movement (REM). Non-REM sleep, which makes up about 75 percent of sleep in adults, has four stages:

Stage 1. The person is relaxing with eyes closed. During this time, respirations are regular, pulse is even, and the person has fleeting thoughts. If awakened, the person will frequently claim he or she had not been sleeping.

Stage 2. It is harder to awaken the person. Fragments of dreams may be experienced, and the eyes may slowly roll from side to side.

Stage 3. The person is very relaxed. Body temperature begins to fall and blood pressure decreases. It is difficult to awaken the person. This stage occurs about twenty minutes after falling asleep.

Stage 4. Deep sleep occurs. The person is very relaxed and responds slowly if awakened.

Approximately ninety minutes into this deep sleep, the human growth hormone, known as somatotropin, is released. Somatotropin's function is to spur the growth of body cells. It acts on the skeleton and skeletal muscles, in particular, to increase their rate of growth and maintain their size and strength. It does this by increasing the rate at which protein enters the cells. Growth hormone also promotes fat-burning by commanding the cells to use fat as energy, and it stimulates cells to release fat to be burned by body cells.

Following stage 4, a sleep pattern of high electrical activity in the brain and deep muscle relaxation, called REM sleep, occurs. Approximately 25 percent of adult sleep is occupied by REM. In contrast, a baby spends up to 50 percent of sleep time in REM. It is my belief that most growth occurs during the REM cycle of sleep. Although it is assumed to be factual information, we have not come across conclusive scientific data to confirm this truth.

It is obvious how important sleep becomes once a person decides to take on an exercise regimen. To facilitate this, it is important to eat protein approximately one and a half to two hours before bedtime and carbohydrates three hours prior to sleep, no less, because sugars and carbohydrates will restrict the function of human growth hormone. You only grow when you sleep, so keep good sleep habits.

I trust this brief journey into the workings of your body will help you understand the necessity of exercise and maintaining a high level of conditioning. The following chapters delve deeper into the digestive process and the importance of proper nutrition.

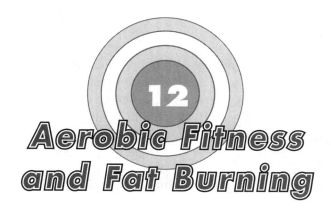

12

Aerobic Fitness and Fat Burning

You can burn a greater amount of fat playing with a yo-yo than climbing a mountain. This may sound preposterous, but it's true. The harder you work at burning fat, the less fat you burn. To understand this concept, you need to understand fat and how it is burned. Fat is actually an incredible substance. It is made by the body and is stored there in times of plenty. Fat has a mind of its own. It loves itself, but is often very lonely and wants plenty of friends. It does not care who you are or what you do. As a matter of fact, it prefers those who do little, and eat a lot. You think fat's bad; fat thinks it's good. *Pile it on* is fat's motto—the more the merrier. Fat loves you and is concerned for your welfare. It believes you're going to starve someday, so it tries to protect you by accumulating deposits around the body. Generally, fat gravitates to areas of little use—fat is a tenant that doesn't like noisy, high-traffic housing. It prefers the quiet life.

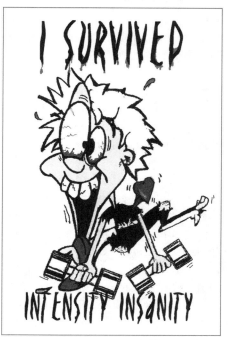

The harder you work . . .
the less fat you burn.

Fat deposits consist of sugars, proteins, and fats that are eaten in excess of your energy output. If you balance input with output, then fat will not accumulate. When you eat more than your body needs, or more than it can process into tissue, that excess is converted into fat. Simply put, fat is stored energy. If you don't burn it, you store it. Energy is the most valuable element in your body. It keeps your heart, lungs, and cells going. It drives the brain, the liver, and so on. Because it is valuable, the body will take every chance it gets to store this energy. But all bodies are not created equal, and some bodies store fat more easily than others. Some bodies have more fat cells and fat-deposit sites than others—it sounds unfair, and it is.

Scientists believe that you accumulate fat-deposit sites, and the number of fat cells in those sites, in the first few years of your life. Others believe genetics are responsible. I feel it's a combination of both—bad luck and bad habits.

The body is always burning fat at some rate, but if your goal is to decrease body fat so lean muscle can show, you have to increase your fat-burning activity. During exercise, the body generally burns carbohydrates for the first twenty minutes. After it has exhausted this reserve of energy, it will go to its alternative source—fat. This is why I believe the first twenty minutes of aerobic exercise is an absolute waste of time. In order to begin burning fat immediately in your cardio routine, you should first do some *anaerobic* activity (weight training). Exercises, such as curls or squats, will exhaust your sugar reserves, thereby allowing you to immediately begin burning fat with your aerobic training. If you burn off the carbohydrates first, then your body will be cocked and ready to burn fat. Once you're in this fat-burning mode, your metabolism will stay elevated, even when the exercise is over.

What is metabolism and why is it important? Metabolism refers to a set of complicated cellular actions that are always running within the body. It's the inner machinery that distributes and regulates body mechanics, such as fat burning, hormone secretion, recovery from illness, respiration, and such. Exercise increases the efficiency of the metabolism. It's a fact that individuals with a high ratio of muscle to fat basically have better metabolisms. This allows for better and more efficient distribution of food.

Muscles are like mini furnaces that burn fat. The more toned a muscle, the more efficient it is at burning fuel, in this case, fat. The argument that you should lose weight before beginning a workout program is preposterous. Nor should the goal ever be just to lose weight. You have some good stuff in there, including bones, muscles, organ tissue, and water. All you want to lose is *excess fat*, not the good stuff. If you attempt aerobics or dieting without toning your body, you will lose muscle. Approximately 20 percent of muscle is lost if you diet or do aerobics alone without weight training. This also equals a 20 percent loss in your ability to burn fat. Therefore, losing weight without toning muscle creates a substantial decrease in fat-burning capacity, and that's not what you want. It is, in fact, the main reason why most diet plans don't work. Yes, you lose weight, and some of that is fat, but a lot of it is good tissue and water.

Although genetics do play a part in your ability to lose or store fat, research shows that anyone can increase his or her metabolism with exercise. Age has little influence on metabolism, except where the muscles have atrophied. Whether you're a senior or an out-of-shape youth, it's the percentage of lean muscle that drives the metabolism. In short, less activity equals less muscle mass, equaling a slower metabolism, equaling increased fat storage and body decay.

There's a lot of confusion regarding the relationship between cardio exercise and fat burning. Let me clear this up for you. If the activity you are performing causes your muscles to exert themselves, you are more than likely burning sugars or carbohydrates instead of fat. If the activity is of low intensity for a prolonged period of time, you will more than likely burn fat.

Heart Rate Formula for Aerobics

To get the maximum benefit from aerobic fitness, it is necessary to maintain a sufficient heart rate that relates specifically to you. To figure this out, the following formula has been developed:

220 – [your age] = 100% of your ideal heart rate

Applying this formula to a forty-year-old, you get 220 – 40 = 180. In this case, 180 beats per minute would be 100 percent of the person's ideal heart rate. Depending on the person's level of fitness, however, a less intense percentage of 60 percent may be desired. In this case, the same formula would apply, but the result would be multiplied by the desired percentage. For example: 220 – 40 = 180. Then, 180 x 0.60 = 108. One hundred and eight beats per minute would then be the targeted heart rate.

For a more accurate reading, a heart monitor is recommended.

This is why: The sugar molecule is small and readily available for transport to a muscle. For example, if you needed to get out of the way of a speeding car fast, the muscles would have to respond quickly. In such a stressful situation, instant energy would be required. And the key here is stress, whether physical or emotional. The harder you work, or the more intense the activity, the more sugar you burn.

Fat is a secondary source of energy. It is a much larger and lazier molecule, and has to be gently coaxed into use. Fat does not respond to stress. This is why you could burn more fat playing with a yo-yo than climbing a mountain. Intensity builds muscle; longevity burns fat. Keys to successful fat burning include the following: First, it is important to change venues for every fat-burning session—use different equipment if available (treadmill, bike, and so on). Second, vary your time and speed at each session. The human body adapts quickly to any kind of activity it does on a regular basis. Some kind of change in fat-burning activity is necessary to fool the body and stay ahead of its ability to adapt.

Here are some helpful answers to the question, "Am I burning fat?":

- If your muscles fatigue during aerobic sessions, you're not burning fat.

- If your muscles are sore after aerobic sessions, you're not burning fat. Muscle fatigue and soreness are indicators that your body is using sugar for energy rather than fat. Soreness indicates the presence of lactic acid, which is partially burned sugar, not fat.

- To be effective, fat burning should seem ridiculously easy.

- Finally, those aerobics classes where everyone moves repetitively in unison, like robots, to the sound of music, are totally useless for burning fat. They burn calories, but not fat.

Aerobic fitness refers to activities that put an oxygen demand on the body. These demands, placed on the body for extended periods of time, will bring about a change in the body's ability to handle oxygen. These changes occur mainly in the lungs, heart, and vascular system. The term *aerobic* means utilization of oxygen, and oxygen is a catalyst for burning fat.

Aerobic fitness is a result of endurance-type activities, which take place over a sustained period of time with an emphasis on breathing. The key to aerobic fitness is not intensity, but duration, a constant, steady pace over time. It's not hard work that counts with aerobic conditioning, it's the building up of endurance over time and distance. When people attempt to make the aerobic exercise more challenging by running or walking up hills, or carrying hand or ankle weights, they are defeating their purpose. The harder the exercise becomes, the more anaerobic it becomes, and while anaerobic exercises do build muscle and bone, they do little for the heart and lungs. They also shut down the fat-burning process for a more efficient source of energy—sugar.

Aerobic activity, combined with a sensible weight-training program, will produce the following results and many, many more. The list is endless.

- Bone and muscle growth

- Emotional relief

- Heart protection

- Higher energy levels

- Improved digestion

- Weight control

Contrary to what people think, aerobics should be a daily commitment. However, if you are also training with the Atomic Fitness System, you can get all the same benefits from thirty to forty minutes of aerobic exercise, three times a week. Outdoor walking or jogging is best, but a stationary bike or treadmill will do just fine. Swimming is also excellent as long as you follow the fat-burning rule: low intensity over a prolonged period of time.

13

Eating Correctly for Fat Reduction

People are not overweight—they are *overfat*. Throw away your scales because weight is irrelevant. It is not your body weight that matters; it's your body fat you should be concerned with.

We are constantly bombarded by advertisements encouraging us to "lose weight," offering some miraculous "weight loss" strategy, and people are tricked into believing this means fat reduction or a thinner waistline. This is simply not true. A lot of products on TV guarantee that you will lose ten pounds in a week. What they're actually doing is giving you a colonic, or diuretic. They're simply cleaning out your insides. You may weigh ten pounds less in a week, but you won't have any change in fat or muscle tone. Your clothes won't fit better . . . you won't look better . . . and certainly, you won't improve your general health. Weight loss could also come from loss of muscle mass. Since muscle mass is what burns body fat, it's apparent you would not want to do that.

The only consideration in losing weight should be in losing fat. A lot of these nonfat products seen on TV, or in the supermarket, are very high in calories and sugar. Sugar converts into fat just as easily as dietary fat turns into fat. Always be conscious of high-glycemic foods (see Table 13.1 on pages 197 and 198) and know the pH levels of what you consume.

The right diet is one that is low in fat and low in fat-converting sugars. It should also be high in protein to maintain muscle tone since muscle is the agent that burns fat. Furthermore, as you'll see, foods should be combined appropriately and eaten at the right intervals.

WHY LOW-CALORIE DIETS DO NOT WORK

The reason you cannot lose weight by starving yourself with a low-calorie diet is because your metabolism will detect any major drop in calories and will then *adjust itself* by burning fewer calories each day.

For example: If you eat 2,500 calories per day, your metabolism will adjust itself so your body burns 2,500 calories per day. If you try to starve yourself by suddenly eating 1,000 calories per day, your metabolism will readjust itself so your body burns only 1,000 calories per day. That's why you have failed in past dieting attempts, and that's why you always seem to fail when you try to starve yourself. Starvation diets promote nothing but indigestion, bloating, and body fat. Weight is gained by eating incorrectly. Weight loss occurs when the right foods are eaten at the right intervals.

FOOD COMBINING

In order to avoid the unpleasant discomforts described above, it is important to adhere to the principles of combining foods properly. There are sound physiological reasons for eating foods in compatible combinations. Some foods will cause digestive distress if mixed together in the digestive system. The principles of food combining are dictated by digestive chemistry. Different foods require different mediums for digestion. Starchy foods, for example, require an alkaline environment for digestion, which is initially supplied in the mouth by the enzyme ptyalin. Protein, on the other hand, requires an acidic medium, such as hydrochloric acid, for proper digestion. As anyone with a basic knowledge of chemistry can tell you, acids and alkalis neutralize each other. If you eat a starch with a protein, digestion will be impaired, if not completely arrested. The food then remains undigested and can cause various digestive problems by becoming a breeding ground for bacteria, which ferment and decompose the food, resulting in a toxic byproduct.

To further illustrate this principle, take the all-American hamburger. The bun is a carbohydrate and the meat is a protein. You consume them together, and they enter the stomach simultaneously. Enzymes turn the food into fluids, and the stomach becomes a holding tank. At this point, it is decided which food will be digested. The body, in a desperate attempt to digest this combination, will leave some undigested food to rot in your stomach, causing bloating, gas, and a swollen lower abdominal region.

The common complaint, particularly with women, is that no matter how much fat they lose, their lower stomach is still in a bloated state, caus-

ing discomfort and looking unfashionable. This is because they have created a constant state of irritable bowel syndrome in their lower tract due to
inefficient eating habits. No amount of exercise will ever flatten a bloated
stomach. The reason is that the internal pressure pushing out from the stomach is greater than the strength of even the strongest abdominal muscles. In
order to avoid this unpleasant condition, it is important to adhere to the following rules of proper food combining:

1. Eat acids (fruits) and starches (pasta, rice) separately. Acids neutralize the
   alkaline environment required for the digestion of starch and result in
   fermentation and indigestion.

2. Eat proteins and carbohydrates at separate meals. Proteins require an
   acidic environment for digestion.

3. Do not eat more than one type of protein per meal.

4. Eat proteins and acidic foods at separate meals. Acidic foods inhibit the
   secretion of the digestive acids required for protein digestion. Undigested protein putrefies in bacterial decomposition and produces some
   potent poisons.

5. Eat fats and proteins at separate meals. Fats slow down the digestive
   process. Some foods, especially nuts with over 50 percent fat, require
   hours for complete digestion.

6. Eat sugars (fruits) and proteins at separate meals.

7. Eat sugars (fruits) and starchy foods at separate meals. Fruits require no
   digestion in the stomach and are held up if they are eaten with foods
   requiring digestion.

8. Eat melons alone. They combine with almost no other food.

9. Skip the desserts. They lie heavy in the stomach, require no digestion,
   and simply ferment.

Foods According to Food Group

The lists of foods in this section will help you get started planning meals
with proper food combinations.

Figure 13.1 further explains which food groups may or may not be combined. The gray arrows show proper food combining, and the black arrows
indicate which food groups should be separated.

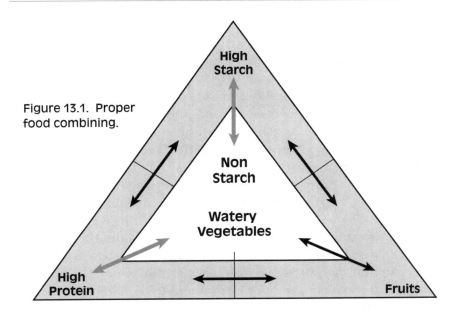

Figure 13.1. Proper food combining.

Foods High in Starch

Avocados
Carrots
Corn
Eggplant
Grains
Pastas
Potatoes (all)
Rice
Squash
Turnips

Non-Starchy Vegetables (High Water Content)

Artichokes
Asparagus
Broccoli
Brussels sprouts
Cabbage
Cauliflower
Celery
Cucumbers
Endive
Green beans
Green leafy
  vegetables
Okra
Parsley
Peppers (all)
Sea vegetables
Swiss chard
Zucchini

Foods High in Protein

Beans
Dairy products
Fish
Legumes
Poultry
Meat (all)
Nuts
Seafood
Seeds
Wild game

Fruits

Apples
Apricots
Bananas
Berries
Cherries
Figs
Grapefruits
Lemons
Melons (all)
Nectarines
Oranges
Peaches
Pears
Pineapples
Plums
Tomatoes

There are also physiological reasons for eating particular food groups at different times of day, as the body's energy requirements vary. For example, in the morning, when you first wake up, the body needs energy. At this point, complex carbohydrates, such as oatmeal, should be taken in. However, the average American breakfast consists of eggs and bacon. The body doesn't need protein in the morning. It needs protein later in the day when it's looking to rebuild. So what happens to the bacon and eggs you've eaten for breakfast? Since the body needs energy at this point, it will take that protein and convert it into sugar to meet its energy requirements. It takes an enormous amount of energy to convert protein into sugar so your body will become even more fatigued rather than energized, and anything left over from the conversion will be stored as fat. The body is being robbed of its energy. This also explains why, by around two to three in the afternoon, most people are falling asleep at their desks. In school, kids are having difficulty concentrating and are not learning. They're all experiencing a tremendous sugar drop, causing their bodies and brains to shut down, all because they've eaten incorrectly. The body is having a hard time rearranging the molecules of food in order to get what it needs.

Therefore, the correct method of eating would be to have carbohydrates in the morning, such as oatmeal or oat products, and avoid eggs and breakfast meats because the body simply doesn't need them. Also it is important to understand that if you are eating carbohydrates, you cannot have caffeine at the same time, due to the fact that caffeine causes fermentation of incompletely digested carbohydrates.

Another popular American breakfast is a buttered roll or a doughnut with a cup of coffee. The coffee impedes the digestion of the buttered roll or doughnut, and raises the blood sugar, causing the inevitable midday crash. The carbohydrates must struggle to get into the body to be stored in the muscle for energy, because most of them will be discharged or stored as fat. It is important to eat your carbohydrates without the caffeine. If you "need" coffee, it should be decaffeinated.

After you've successfully eaten your carbohydrates, you should have a protein meal two to three hours later, and it should consist solely of one kind of protein. Egg whites, chicken, turkey, lean red meats, and fish are all good choices. (Note, though, that many types of fish are now considered toxic, so it is necessary to choose carefully among the remaining varieties considered safe.) If you are a vegetarian, you may consider soybeans and tofu. Greens such as asparagus, broccoli, romaine lettuce, and spinach may also be eaten at this time, before your protein. These are very good sources of enzymes and phytonutrients. Two or three hours after your protein meal, you should have a small snack, such as fruit. Fruit requires little digestion and should be eaten alone.

Remember, don't eat foods that require digestion with those that require none. The food that requires little digestion will sit in the stomach and rot. Again, this will result in bloating, gas, discomfort, and an imbalance in your pH level.

The last meal of the day should be a light protein meal of some sort. During the night, specifically one and a half hours into sleep, the human body rebuilds all tissue. Then, about one and a half hours before awakening, the body shuts down this mechanism and goes into energy production.

ENERGY AND ITS RELATIONSHIP TO BEING OVERWEIGHT AND FAT

In the beginning, we were all created equal, but life and evolution changed that. If your ancestors lived in caves, you most likely have trouble losing fat. Your ancestors had to hide in caves to stay alive. The harsh weather conditions and the danger of being killed kept some early humans sheltered for long periods of time. This inability to hunt every day and have sufficient energy supplies caused some to develop the ability to store food as energy in the form of fat as a means of staying alive during famine. Although it has been a long time since humans lived in caves, this condition still exists today.

There are others, however, whose ancestors roamed the lands in a never-ending cycle of hunting, eating, and camping. These ancient relatives produced offspring that did not store energy, for food was plenty. Today, these individuals have a natural tendency to be muscular and lean.

You should understand that fat is basically stored energy. You *get* fat when you've consumed more energy than your body is able to use. Although sugar is the primary source of energy for the body, and the preferred source of quick energy for the muscles, the main source of long-term energy is fat.

Just as gas is to an engine, fat and sugar are to the human body, and just as people value gold, diamonds, and precious jewels, the human body values sugar. Once the human body recognizes sugar, it does not want to let it go. Unfortunately, it has a limited capacity to store sugar, so any excess sugar it cannot use for energy is converted into a substance it can store in abundance—fat. Fat, as I said, is simply stored energy.

As an energy supply, sugar is very valuable. The body can store some sugar in the liver and some in the muscle, but after that, the overflow goes into the bloodstream to be converted and stored as fat because the body does not want to lose this valuable energy supply. The body has the ability to carry two, three, even four hundred pounds of fat, or blubber. It is a glutton for this gold, this precious jewel, this sugar, and it doesn't like to let it go. That's why it is so difficult to lose fat. The body is reluctant to part with it, and quite literally, it has to be tricked into giving its fat supply up.

Exercise plays a major role in the burning of fat. Eating correctly plays a major role in assuring that it is not replaced. Most people who diet without exercising do not understand they're not just losing fat, they're also losing muscle. Since muscle is responsible for burning fat, they're creating a catch-22 situation for themselves. Although dieting alone may seem to be effective at first, the decrease in muscle that accompanies the initial weight loss will make it increasingly more difficult to shed additional fat reserves. This point cannot be overemphasized—decrease your muscle, decrease your ability to burn fat.

Let me reiterate how important proper food combining is to weight loss. A subtle but common mistake many people make is to eat two sources of energy at the same time, such as putting butter on their corn. Corn is a simple sugar and butter is a fat. You've now created a situation in which your body is consuming two sources of energy. It will first use the simple sugar for energy and automatically store the fat as surplus energy.

Foods that are high on the glycemic index (those that cause a fast rise in blood sugar; see Table 13.1) are more fattening than fatty foods. It may seem strange to think of a carrot as more fattening than butter, but the reasoning behind this theory is that the fat in the butter does not adversely affect insulin levels, whereas the high concentration of sugar in the carrot plays tricks on the endocrine system, causing insulin levels to spike and sugar levels to drop. The body equates this sudden drop in blood sugar with low energy, and believes it has no energy left. The body then sends a message to the digestive tract to absorb and store everything in it, thereby turning everything to fat. This is true even with a 400-pound man. The body doesn't determine its needs by reading body fat. Messages are sent through the bloodstream.

Let's take another look at the American diet: A couple goes out to dinner. The waiter asks if he can get them something from the bar. Alcohol, which is super high on the glycemic index, hits the bloodstream and signals the production of insulin to get rid of the sugar. The insulin lowers the blood sugar level to a point where the body thinks it doesn't have enough sugar

TABLE 13.1. GLYCEMIC INDEX

Cereals	
All-Bran	51
All-Bran Buds + psyllium	45
Bran Flakes	74
Cheerios	74
Corn Chex	83
Cornflakes	83
Cream of Wheat	66
Frosted Flakes	55
Grapenuts	67
Life Cereal	66
Muesli, natural	54
Nutri-grain	66
Oatmeal, old fashioned	48
Puffed Wheat	67
Raisin Bran	73
Rice Chex	89
Shredded Wheat	67
Special K	54
Total Cereal	76

Fruit	
apple	38
apricots	57
banana	56
cantalope	65
cherries	22
dates	103
grapefruit	25
grapes	46
kiwi	52
mango	55
orange	43
papaya	58
peach	42
pear	58
pineapple	66
plums	39
prunes	15
raisins	64
watermelon	72

Snacks	
chocolate bar	49
corn chips	72
croissant	67
doughnut	76
jelly beans	80
Life Savers	70
oatmeal cookie	57
pizza, cheese & tomatoes	60
Pizza Hut, supreme	33
popcorn, light microwave	55
potato chips	56
pound cake	54
Power bars	58
pretzels	83
shortbread cookies	64
Snikers bar	41
strawberry jam	51
vanilla wafers	77

Crackers	
graham crackers	74
rice cakes	80
rye	68
saltine crackers	74
soda crackers	72
Wheat Thins	67

Cereal Grains	
barley	25
basmati white rice	58
bulgar	48
couscous	65
cornmeal	68
millet	71

Sugars	
fructose	22
honey	62
maltose	105
table sugar	64

Pasta	
cheese tortellini	50
fettucini	32
linguini	50
macaroni	46
spaghetti, 5-minutes boiled	33
spaghetti, 15-minutes boiled	44
spaghetti, protein-enriched	28
vermicelli	35

Soups/Vegetables

beets, canned	64
black bean soup	64
carrots, fresh, boiled	49
corn, sweet	56
green pea soup	66
green peas, frozen	47
lima beans, frozen	32
parsnips	97
peas, fresh, boiled	48
split-pea soup w/ham	66
tomato soup	38

Drinks

apple juice	40
colas	65
Gatorade	78
grapefruit juice	48
orange juice	46
pineapple juice	46

Milk Products

chocolate milk	35
custard	43
ice cream, vanilla	60
ice milk, vanilla	50
skim milk	32
soy milk	31
tofu frozen dessert	115
whole milk	30
yogurt, w/fruit	36
yogurt, plain	14

Beans

baked beans	44
black beans, boiled	30
butter beans, boiled	33
cannellini beans	31
garbanzos, boiled	34
kidney beans, boiled	29
kidney beans, canned	52
lentils, green, brown	30
lima beans, boiled	32
navy beans	38
pinto beans, boiled	39
red lentils, boiled	27
soybeans, boiled	16

Breads

bagel, plain	72
baquette, French	95
croissant	67
dark rye	76
hamburger bun	61

Muffins

apple, cinnamon	44
blueberry	59
oat & raisin	54
pita	57
pizza, cheese	60
pumpernickel	49
sourdough	54
rye	64
white	70
wheat	68

Root Crops

french fries	75
potatoes, new, boiled	59
potatoes, red, baked	93
potatoes, sweet	52
potatoes, white, boiled	63
potatoes, white, mash	70
yam	54

and the body goes into energy debt. The body is now convinced that everything it takes in from this point on must be reserved for energy and converted to fat. And this is accompanied by a false sense of hunger because the body thinks it needs food.

So, here are these people drinking high-glycemic-index beverages at the beginning of the meal, setting up everything else they eat from then on to become storage. There's little chance any of it will be used as energy, and even less chance it will be used as building material, because the body hormones, which are messengers from the endocrine system, are telling the body to store the food as fat for emergency measures.

On top of that, the couple is having wine and salad, which could contain beets, carrots, cauliflower, or tomatoes, all high in sugar. Now the body has another message, just in case it missed the first one, to make sure everything taken in is stored as fat.

Then comes the main course. It's protein, but not just protein. The side dishes consist of starches—potatoes or pasta—more carbohydrates and sugar. And don't even discuss the desserts. So, the couple goes home, and for the next twenty-four hours the fat-storage system they've established stays in gear. Their bodies are robbed of energy because it's all been used up creating storage reserves. They think they're hungry, so they have a snack. The body becomes so bogged down with carbohydrate storage that they're not even able to digest and utilize the protein they had.

Since most of America today is doing 100 percent of the wrong thing 100

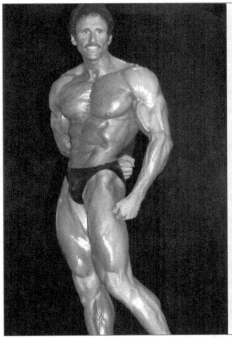
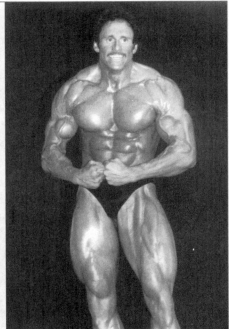

It takes incredible knowledge of all the sciences to build a body like this.

The proof is in the results.

percent of the time, if you can achieve as little as a 20 percent change in your diet, you'll be 20 percent ahead . . . 50 percent, 50 percent ahead . . . 80 percent, 80 percent ahead. Nobody expects you to be 100 percent perfect 100 percent of the time, but you'll certainly look and feel a lot better if you apply the basic premises and principles I've laid out in this chapter.

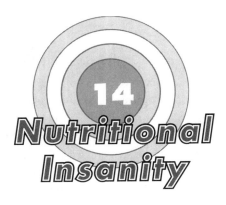

14

Nutritional Insanity

The Macrobiotic Diet, Atkins, Pritikin, the Zone Diet, the Blood Type Diet—it's all enough to make you crazy. It makes me a bit crazy, too. Today, we have several competing and conflicting diets, each of which must work for some or they never would have gotten off the ground. Yet, none of them work for everyone. How does one make sense of it all?

In the 1980s, I became aware of work being done with pH levels. The research was based on the principle that meat and protein cause the body to acidify, and fruits and vegetables make the body more alkaline. It was discovered that when a diet was altered to complement an individual's metabolism, the pH levels were brought into proper balance and the person lost body fat. The tests showed how subtle shifts with diet and supplements could normalize pH and raise body metabolism, thus aiding fat loss.

In his book, *The Metabolic Typing Diet*, William Wolcott explains his dominance theory of individual metabolism. He describes two competing factors of metabolism in the body: the autonomic (unconscious) nervous system (ANS) and the oxidative system. In each, foods and nutrients have opposing effects on a body's pH level. For example, it is generally known that potassium and magnesium are alkalinizing—or are they? In reality, this is determined by which of the two systems is dominant in an individual.

The autonomic system has two parts, the sympathetic, which activates the metabolism, and the parasympathetic, which slows the metabolism down. The latter controls digestion, tends to unwind the system, and promotes alkalinization of the body when it's active. The sympathetic branch winds you up, gets adrenaline pumping, and tends to acidify the body when active, increasing the metabolic process.

Therefore, according to Wolcott, "The net effect of pH depends on which system is dominant in the given individual." All of a sudden, it makes sense how and why one diet may work so well for one person yet fail miserably for another. With today's epidemic of obesity, knowing your metabolic type is extremely important. For example, if you have a parasympathetic dominance and are already alkaline, eating foods that further stimulate the parasympathetic system (carbohydrates and sugars—a vegetarian-based diet) will only push you into further imbalance. If, on the other hand, you are oxidative dominant and a slow oxidizer, your system will be balanced by a vegetarian-based diet. It will provide the vitamins and minerals you need to speed up oxidation and generate more acids to balance you out. (*See* Appendix A for a listing of alkalizing and acidifying foods.)

How do you know what type of metabolism you have? First, to make it simpler, understand that there are essentially four metabolic types: pro-metabolic, anti-metabolic, oxidative-fast, and oxidative-slow. However, there are only two basic diets. This makes it even easier. The degree of adherence is determined by how dominant a system (for example, the oxidative system) is in your body. Oxidative-fast and anti-metabolism types fall into the group A category. Carbohydrate-rich diets tend to be detrimental for this group whose diets should lean toward proteins and fats as preferred fuel sources. Pro-metabolic and oxidative-slow types are in group B, and they possess a greater tolerance for carbohydrates. Group B diets should be more heavily weighted toward light, non-fatty proteins, with an abundance of vegetables. Neither group should ever be eating refined carbohydrates (starch and sugar). Carbohydrates that are refined are dead food. Dead is dead and can only build toxins, not give life to your cells. Some people are blessed to be balanced and have much greater dietary freedom.

A quick way to determine your metabolic type is to take a fasting glucose blood test, or a triglycerides (fats) test. While the reference range for insulin may go from 0 to 160, it is the general belief that any value over 80 suggests excessive insulin activity; that is, too many carbohydrates are being converted into fats. As the numbers increase, so does this condition. People who fall into this category would most likely do well on a group A diet, or a low-carbohydrate diet.

For those with triglycerides lower than 80, a simple test to gauge pH and blood sugar response to a glucose challenge can identify your type. This metabolic-type testing is unnecessary if either your triglycerides or fasting glucose is high, since you already know that your body will do much better with very few carbohydrates. (Unfortunately, while good in times of

Toxic Fat Response

If you accumulate enough toxins in your body from food allergies or from food you are sensitive to, you will store body fat more easily. Certain foods trigger this toxic fat response. The body perceives these foods as invaders, increasing your white blood cell count, which triggers your immune system because the food is identified as a foreign invader. This triggering of the immune response disrupts normal metabolic activities and doesn't allow food to be processed, so it's stored as fat. Research has shown that such toxic foods can adversely affect brain chemistry and can actually result in a false craving for these toxic foods.

Once the immune system responds to what it believes to be harmful to the body, it will create specific antibodies. As these antibodies grow, your immune system will release body chemicals in order to protect itself. Unfortunately, these chemicals have an adverse effect on your body, causing problems in the gastrointestinal tract, respiratory and cardiovascular malfunction, and can lead to obesity and even death.

From bodybuilders to homemakers, anyone who is interested in reducing water retention or bloating should heed the fact that toxic foods will trigger bloating in the lower abdominal area, and no amount of exercise or starvation dieting will remedy this condition. Up to 40 percent of your body weight can be attributed to the intake of toxic foods. Excess fluid will leak out from your stomach and intestines onto the skin, giving you the appearance of body fat, bloating in the face, and filling out the curvature of your body, which can detract from your appearance. No exercise will help this; no calorie restriction can remedy this; no Atkins or Zone diet, and so on, will have any effect on this condition. The only solution is to avoid the foods that are toxic to your system.

Although many foods can be toxic depending on the individual, the most common toxic foods are eggs, fish, milk (cow's and goat's), peanuts, shellfish, soy, tree nuts (cashews and walnuts), and wheat products. Be aware that many foods contain one or more of these substances.

famine, your system can be very troublesome in times of plenty.) This takes a lot of the guesswork out of dieting. Furthermore, the testing can identify those headed toward obesity long in advance.

Some people possess a thrifty gene that stores fuel to spare the body in times of famine. Hundreds of years ago, when food supplies were scarce, this gene served a critical function. It kept those who possessed it alive. Today, however, particularly in the United States where food supplies are plenty, people with this gene continue to store everything they eat, eventually leading to obesity. The gene works through the overproduction of insulin, which quickly clears blood sugar (from carbohydrates), converting the glucose to triglycerides and fats for storage. As long as insulin is around, carbohydrates are headed into the fat-for-storage depot. The only significant stimulus for insulin is the ingestion of carbohydrates, with *refined* carbohydrates and sugars being the worst of the insulin stimulators. The body has a hatred for high blood sugar since it causes damage to blood vessels.

In addition to this unbroken chain of food storage leading to pathologic obesity, such high levels of insulin can cause an undesirable medical condition most commonly known as Syndrome X. High insulin is one of the biggest risk factors for the inability to lose weight. It causes depositions of fat all over the body, fatigue, fluid retention, and may directly age DNA (genetic material), possibly making it one of the greatest aging factors. Low insulin, on the other hand, slows the aging of DNA and maximizes lifespan. By burning fuel rather than calling on insulin to store it, exercise, like calorie and carbohydrate restriction, helps get rid of the fat-storing insulin—provided you do not compensate by ingesting more carbohydrates.

We all have different metabolisms, which is why one diet works for some but not others, and why the Atomic Fitness Nutrition Plan applies to everyone (see Chapter 15). Once you determine your metabolic type, you can balance your meals accordingly. Once you eat a diet right for your system, and avoid refined carbohydrates and calories with a high-glycemic value, you should lose fat.

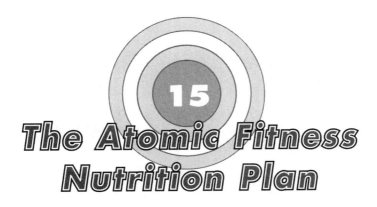

The Atomic Fitness Nutrition Plan

15

The Atomic Fitness Nutrition Plan is a commonsense approach to eating based on the biological factors of the human body. This plan applies to those who want to gain lean mass and those who want to lose body fat. The only difference is the amount of food eaten and how many times you eat.

Quite frankly, unless I were to meet you in person, it would be impossible to design a nutritional program that addresses your individual needs. Every body has unique physiological and psychological properties that determine how food is utilized, as well as where fat is stored, and how the body uses nutrition to build muscle. Lifestyle and socioeconomic conditions are also factors. This is why I advocate teaching you the basic, standard rules you need to obtain optimal results.

The truth of the matter is there's no need to follow some complicated dietary formula or starve yourself with tasteless foods. All that is necessary is to follow the basic guidelines set forth by the Atomic Fitness Nutrition Plan and let exercise do the rest.

GUIDELINES FOR THE ATOMIC FITNESS NUTRITIONAL PLAN

The following sixteen points constitute the core rules of the Atomic Fitness Nutrition Plan.

1. Food groups should be eaten separately at different meals. It is critical that you separate proteins and carbohydrates, especially those consisting of starches and sugars, to allow for proper digestion and to avoid

bloating. Also, meals should be eaten no closer than two hours apart. Do not eat more than one type of protein per meal.

2. The only exception to rule #1 is that green leafy vegetables, such as spinach and romaine lettuce, may be eaten with protein in the same meal without interfering with the digestion of either.

3. Limit your intake of high-glycemic carbohydrates. Carbohydrates, such as oatmeal, with glycemic counts of 60 and below are good choices. (See Table 13.1 on pages 197–198 for further information.)

4. Limit fats to essential (good) fats, such as almonds and salmon. (*See* the section on fats in Chapter 16 for further information.)

5. Increase dairy for calcium requirements. Good choices include low-fat milk, low-fat yogurt, low-fat cheese (not milled), and so on.

6. Mornings should consist of nutrient-dense, high-fiber carbohydrates. Good choices include oatmeal or other whole-grain oats—not wheat or corn.

7. Limit salt intake. According to the U.S. Department of Health and Human Services, the daily salt allowance should not exceed 2,400 milligrams per day. That is the approximate equivalent of one teaspoon of table salt. Read your labels.

8. It is important to drink lots of water. It is recommended that the average person drink at least eight glasses a day. More may be required, depending on your level of activity. If you feel thirsty, you're already dehydrated.

9. Fruits should not be eaten with other food. Since fruit requires relatively no time for digestion, it may be eaten as little as a half hour prior to meals. However, after a meal, to ensure proper digestion of the other nutrients, you should wait two hours before eating fruit.

10. To maintain lean mass and lose body fat, it is recommended that you take in 1 gram of protein per pound of body weight. For example, if you weigh 120 pounds, you should take in 120 grams of protein each day.

11. To gain lean mass, it is recommended that you take in 2 grams of protein per pound of body weight. For example, if you weigh 120 pounds, you should take in 240 grams of protein each day.

12. On training days, add one piece of fruit immediately following your workout. This simple carbohydrate spares precious protein for muscle building. The muscles will use the carbohydrates from the fruit for recovery instead.

13. Caffeinated beverages should be limited to three cups a day.

14. Refrain from consuming hard liquor. Beer and wine are acceptable on cheat day only (*see* #16). If you must consume beer or wine on your cheat day, limit yourself to two beers or one glass of wine.

15. Individual requirements regarding carbohydrates vary. Everyone's needs are different. Follow the Atomic Fitness Nutrition Plan, using experimentation if necessary, to find your personal optimum level of intake.

16. Take a cheat day once a week. This is the day to satisfy your cravings. It's okay. It won't hurt you. There are no limits on the types of foods you eat on this day, only the amounts. Eat the same number of meals, in the same proportions you normally would, but, for example, replace the apple with a scoop of ice cream.

   Here's how the cheat day works: For six days, you're eating a consistent pattern of similar foods. Your body begins to recognize this pattern and establishes the required mechanisms (enzymes) to digest the foods it has become accustomed to. On the seventh day, however, if you eat foods the body is not accustomed to, the mechanisms (enzymes) will not be available to assimilate these unfamiliar substances into the body. In effect, your body will not recognize the ice cream you just ate as food, so the body will simply pass it through your system without absorbing it or turning it into fat. For this to work effectively, it is important that you designate, and maintain, the same cheat day each week. For example, if you decide your cheat day will be Sunday, it must remain Sunday. It can't be Sunday one week and Wednesday the next.

Now that you are armed with the basic guidelines of the nutrition plan, let's get down to some specifics.

SAMPLE EATING SCHEDULE

The following eating schedule outlines what foods are appropriate for specific times of day and lists good times to eat for proper digestion.

7 A.M.

Breakfast: Low-glycemic, nutrient-dense carbohydrates (oatmeal or other whole-grain oat products, or rye—avoid corn or wheat)

10 A.M.

Mid-morning snack: Protein (chicken, egg whites, and fish)

    Females: 25 grams (approximately 4 ounces)

    Males: 50 grams (approximately 8 ounces)

There should be no more than three hours between the mid-morning snack and lunch.

1 P.M.

Lunch: Protein and green leafy vegetables

There should be no more than two hours between lunch and the mid-afternoon snack.

3 P.M.

Mid-afternoon snack: Piece of fruit

There should be more than three hours between the mid-afternoon snack and dinner.

6 P.M.

Dinner: Protein and green leafy vegetables

Do not eat after 7 P.M.

    Note: Hunger is *not* an indication that your body needs more food. It's an indication that your stomach is shrinking. If you experience hunger between meals, *drink water.*

SUGGESTED DIET TO REDUCE BODY FAT

The following system of eating may be used to train the liver to access and utilize the body's fat supply for energy, rather than using sugar and carbohydrates. The obvious benefits of this are a reduction of fat reserves, resulting in leaner body mass. Also, by using fat for energy, rather than sugar and carbohydrates, you increase your stamina. This is due to the fact that energy is based on calories. One gram of fat has double the calories of sugar. Fat is also a slower-releasing energy source. Therefore, you can do twice the work if you're using fat for energy rather than carbohydrates or sugar.

The following dietary system is based on cycles of days. This system adjusts the body to dietary changes gradually in order to avoid shocking the body and causing any adverse side affects.

Caution: It is important that anyone with health concerns, such as diabetes, avoid this diet.

Cycle 1

Start by eating only protein for two consecutive days. On protein days, it is critical to keep your intake of carbohydrates as close to zero as possible.

On the third day, eat only carbohydrates. Try to confine yourself to healthy complex carbohydrates, such as fruits, oatmeal, vegetables, and whole grains.

On days four and five, you will return to eating only protein, followed again by a day of carbohydrates.

This pattern should continue for a cycle of twelve to eighteen days.

Cycle 2

Following your last day of carbohydrates on cycle 1, increase your protein days to three consecutive days, followed again by one day of carbohydrates.

This cycle should continue for approximately one month.

Cycle 3

Following your last day of carbohydrates on cycle 2, increase your protein days to four consecutive days, followed once more by one day of carbohydrates.

Continue cycle 3 for approximately two weeks before moving on to the final cycle.

Cycle 4

During this last cycle, you will increase your protein days to six consecutive days and you will complete this cycle with one cheat day. On this day, you are allowed to eat absolutely anything you desire, provided you do not increase your proportions or the number of meals. As explained, your body will not recognize the foreign substances you're ingesting and will not, therefore, have the necessary enzymes available to assimilate them into your system. Your cheat day will not make you fat, and it will help you maintain your discipline by giving you a reward to look forward to.

This final cycle only requires one week, making it necessary to complete only one phase of cycle 4.

You're done.

Upon completion of this pattern of cycles, assess your fat loss. Do *not* use a scale. Scales do not weigh fat. Simply look in the mirror. See how your clothes fit. Are you happy with the level of fat reduction you've achieved? If so, you have successfully completed the metabolic correction diet and your liver is now processing fats and protein into energy. In order to maintain this desirable condition, you should adhere to the basic guidelines outlined in the Atomic Fitness Nutrition Plan.

If you are not satisfied with your results and feel you have additional fat that needs to be reduced, repeat the system of cycling from the top until you have attained your desired goal.

The metabolic correction diet is designed to kick-start your fat-burning metabolism in record time. The system efficiently switches your body into a fat-burning unit while correcting blood sugar levels and balancing out hypoglycemic episodes, thereby eliminating mood swings, giving you more energy, and allowing you to think more clearly.

Cravings and hunger become almost nonexistent. Your desire for the kinds of destructive foods you've consumed in the past will disappear.

Your cheat day, a reward day, gives you something to look forward to. You will see results and be happy to continue.

With this cycle, you will be geared to create a positive metabolic balance that will enhance muscle growth and promote fat burning. As great as it is, however, it is *only* to be used to kick-start your system into rocket progress. It is not a lifetime or lifestyle change. Healthy long-term dieting should follow the basic rules for good eating that are provided in the Atomic Fitness Nutrition Plan guidelines and eating schedule. In the following chapter, I will go into more detail about food, nutrition, and the digestive process so that you can better understand how to maintain healthy eating for life.

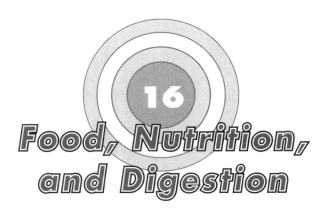

16
Food, Nutrition, and Digestion

It is well established that proper eating allows you to do more and to be a better competitor. Your diet needs to meet both your energy demands and nutritional requirements and will be effective only when it meets all the various demands placed on it through physical activity. If these demands are not fulfilled through diet, you can easily become extremely fatigued.

As elite athletes know, skill and physical training are just not enough

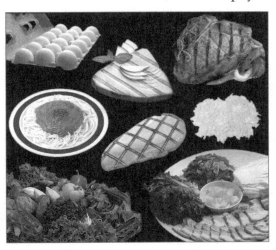

for the competitive edge. Athletes have specific dietary needs, and an integration of all available training technologies, including proper nutrition, contributes significantly to peak performance.

A proper combination of food types is critical to supplying ample energy for your particular physical demands and recovery needs. Not all athletes require the same nutrition, but without good nutrition and proper supplementation, you will find it difficult to improve on your physical performance.

There are six major nutrients essential to healthy living and prosperous athletic pursuits. These include carbohydrates, fats, minerals, proteins, vitamins, and water. A deficiency in any of these major nutrients can leave you performing at less than your full potential.

FOOD AND EXERCISE

You must find out what the body wants and needs from you. Keep in mind that the body wants to achieve a balance (homeostasis) of its cells, hormones, and structure. How do you start? First, you must learn the basic fundamentals of eating. With every bite of food, every intake of fluids, and every breath, you're signaling the body to go in and out of homeostasis.

Eating food in the proper combinations and in a controlled way is your ticket to balance. Staying in balance is a matter of knowing the rules and principles the body must follow, and following them. Basically, the human body does not think, it reacts. It does not lead, it follows the orders you give it, some of which are given every time you eat or drink. Like any other machine, the body needs an endless supply of energy and building blocks. A lean, muscular body, produced by eating correctly, will allow you to achieve this. It's simple. If you follow the rules, you win. If you eat the wrong foods at the wrong times and in the incorrect proportions, you lose.

Mainstream dietitians, doctors, and nutritionists are well-intended but ill-informed, and they can often steer you down the pathway to destruction. If you want to increase the efficiency of your life, and have a stronger, healthier body and mind, stay out of this maze of misinformation.

The way people eat is sometimes governed by fads or miracle diets, usually promoted by self-proclaimed diet experts who announce scientific diet breakthroughs based on incorrect information. In addition, the government standard for eating correctly has been dead wrong for years. You've been deceived by balance-your-plate diets, containing all the food groups in one meal, that violate the basic physiology of digestion.

The rule of reason and understanding has been replaced by confusion and frustration. People have gotten to the point where they are desperate, and desperation leads to apathy. However, there is a message of hope here: if you learn how mainstream diets are harmful, then you are on your way to providing your body with the nutrients it needs for a lifetime of health.

Let's take another look at how people eat. In our society, people eat feed, the same feed that is served to livestock, such as cows and pigs. They are fed grains, potatoes, and rice to fatten them up. Sound familiar? It should. It's the same diet the government-sponsored food pyramid recommends for the human population. People in the United States have been duped into eating like cows, with diets that consist of flour products, grains, and a class of protein the body can only absorb as fat. And don't be fooled by packages advertising that the product is fat-free. Read the label, for it is sure to be high in carbohydrates. Look around you. This is a country shaped like, and acting like, livestock—fat and lethargic. This country has spent billions on healthcare, trillions on research, and it is still the fattest and most out-of-shape culture on Earth. Something just doesn't add up.

Leading authorities have said that a high-protein diet is unnecessary, that fat in your diet will kill you, and that a high-carbohydrate diet is ideal. For over two decades, leading food-industry advertisers have brainwashed people into believing that the low-fat carbohydrate diet is the healthiest for you. If this is the case, why is it that over the years there has been an increase in cases of arthritis, cancer, cardiovascular disease, diabetes, heart disease, and other diet-related diseases? There are also these fad diets that simply don't work, such as the cabbage diet where you eat nothing but cabbage. Then there's the "drink-water-a-billion-times-a-day" diet. And diets featuring bars, creams, colonics, diuretics, pills, shakes, plus the Hollywood diet or the Subway diet, and so on, will just lead you straight down the pathway to disaster. Out-of-shape bodies with unbalanced body chemistries have become an epidemic in this society.

It's time to open your eyes and your mind. You can start by examining what you eat and how it affects you. The following are some basics you should know.

- You will not lose weight by starving yourself. This diet will only serve to slow down your metabolism. It will lead to muscle and bone loss, and you will simply become fatigued and fatter—not a good scenario. Every time you lower your caloric intake, your body will slow down its metabolism to compensate.

- Another myth is that all fats are bad for you. This is not true. There are necessary good fats that should be part of your diet. These fats will actually help clean out bad body fats. Also, a low-fat diet triggers a scarcity of fat in the body, which leads to excess fat storage. The body will also convert other foods to fat in a desperate attempt to supplement the proper amount of missing fat. Don't be afraid of good fats like fish oil, flaxseed, and conjugated linoleic acid (CLA).

Food is a controlling factor for the body. Eating correctly in the right combinations, and understanding the principles of digestion and how those principles affect your emotions (via the hormones) will go a long way toward maintaining your life and happiness.

Let's make a simple comparison to a computer, with food as the software and the body as the hardware. Putting in a certain type of food is like installing a particular program. The food will stimulate certain hormones, which will affect how it plays out in your body. Each food runs a different program, and different combinations of food will cause different effects. What you put in your mouth with your own hand will determine your fate. The human machine can endure most anything, and it will try in desperation to adapt to the worst conditions. It is this adaptation that uses up so much of the body's energy and can leave you tired and confused.

How then to get on the path to a power-packed, muscular body? One of the first steps is through *proper* nutrition. Knowing how to control the three macronutrients—carbohydrates, fats, and proteins—is the gateway to the real power. You can achieve this by studying, and understanding, the macronutrients and how they interrelate with the body and each other. These nutrients generate a hormonal response that can affect how people act, feel, and think because hormones are the command centers of the body. They regulate almost all functions, and staying strong and lean means keeping the body's key hormone levels in balance.

The reality is that the best and most complete digestion takes place when there is only one food group in the digestive system, as opposed to a variety. This was discussed previously, but I can't stress it enough. The digestive tract will vary its enzymes and fluids according to what foods are present. In order for foods to be more easily digested and absorbed, these variations must include the changes in fluid pH levels. Different foods require different pH environments, either acidic or alkaline. If you mix acids and alkalis together, they counter each other's efficiency and potency. Have you ever seen the old magic trick where the magician pours blue fluids (acids) into a cup of red fluid (alkali) and it all turns clear? When you mix an acid with an alkali, it turns to water. And food *cannot* digest in water. Therefore, attempting to exercise or train with a stomach of partially digested, mixed acidic and alkaline foods is certainly a less-than-optimum situation. This causes bloating, gas, and indigestion, and will rob you of energy, even make you ill.

The timing and amounts of concentrated enzymes being released is also affected by the types of food eaten. Matching fluids and enzymes to the type of food eaten is critical, and this can only work properly when the characteristics of the foods eaten are similar to one another. Dissimilar foods, such as bread and cheese, disrupt the efficiency of the digestive system. Natural food combinations that contain both protein and carbohydrates, as in some whole grains, are digested more easily because nature has provided enzymes in the food to aid the digestive system. It is the more prevalent food combinations, such as meat and flour as in the sandwich, that cause most of the problems. You will never get rid of that potbelly or bloating if you don't understand this basic premise.

In a sense, the body is subjected to digestive poisoning when foods are mixed incorrectly. In this way, food can truly corrupt the body and mind. Most people do not eat one food type at a time (per meal). They don't eat, for example, the meat, then follow it with the carbohydrates or the starch. They eat these foods together, as with eggs and toast, meat and potatoes, or a sandwich. Tests have shown a large amount of undigested starch in the stools of people who mix their protein and carbohydrates together, indicating the inability of the body to digest these macronutrients together. Undigested food wastes both energy and nutrients.

Proteins digest best in a high-acid environment, while carbohydrates prefer one that is more alkaline. It stands to reason then that the best meals are the simplest ones, where the macronutrients are separated.

I wish to again review the absorption, digestion, and utilization of food. Food is governed by the laws of science and chemistry. Protein digestion requires an acidic environment. Starch digestion requires an alkaline environment. Sugar does best with a lactose-type enzyme, and none of these work well together. Sometimes, they will even cancel one another out, leaving food to digest in a watery fluid base. Food left in water will rot. It is just a matter of chemistry—rotted food is a garbage dump, a cesspool of filth and disease, and it's inside you.

People take indigestion for granted. Bloating, gas, stomach pains, and so forth are considered normal, but they're not. They are real danger signals. How does society handle these danger signals? With Alka-Seltzer, Pepto-Bismol, or Tums. Wake up, you're killing yourself, and the pharmaceutical industry is making a fortune from your ignorance.

Take a cue from the animal kingdom. Animals will only eat one food type at a time. You'll never see a lion eat an antelope and then some shrubs. In general, the animal kingdom follows the natural laws of eating, and sickness is rare. On the other hand, humans, in their ultimate wisdom, have created the sandwich.

Digestion is the act of breaking down food to obtain its energies. These energies are vital to your well-being and performance in life. You are what you consume. If you don't consume correctly, you will *be consumed*. Many die of hunger, many more die from eating.

Eating too much is equally destructive. Consuming more than the body can use leads to indigestion and gastric diseases. Advertisers clearly have been successful in convincing people that their eyes are big enough for their mouths because, too often, everything people see, they eat. The solution to this is simple: eat smaller portions more often. This leads to the next issue, regularity—the best time, and how often, to eat.

Most people eat whenever they find time within the framework of a three-meal day, but it is ideal to eat with regularity, at the same time every day, and in small amounts, altering the type of food eaten at each meal. For example, if the first meal is a carbohydrate, then the next meal should be protein, followed by another carbohydrate meal, and so on, alternating meals in this way, unless otherwise specified in this text. For guidance, refer to the sample meal schedule in Chapter 15.

All of nature works through cycles or rhythms, including the human body. Unfortunately though, the only rhythm man has developed is hunger and gluttony. The rhythms of the body tie into everything. The digestive rhythms have a limited supply of digestive enzymes flowing, and they have their maximum effect and are in greater amounts while eating. After eating, they are in very limited supply, so time between meals must be allotted for the digestive system to kick in again. A bogged-down, slow-moving digestive tract will cause food to rot and ferment before it is eliminated. Do you honestly believe a body filled with waste will help you be your best? Think about it.

METABOLISM

Metabolism refers to all the chemical reactions of the body. The body's metabolism may be thought of as an energy-balancing act between catabolic (breaking down) reactions, which provide energy, and anabolic reactions (building up), which require energy.

Catabolism is the term for decompositional chemical reactions that provide energy. Digestion is a catabolic process in which the breaking down of food molecules releases energy. Oxidation, also a catabolic process, is the removal of electrons and hydrogen from a molecule, or less frequently, the addition of oxygen to a molecule. Glucose is the body's favorite nutrient for oxidation, but fats and proteins are also oxidized. As substances are oxidized, energy is produced.

The opposite of catabolism is anabolism. Anabolism is a series of reactions whereby small molecules are built up into larger ones that form the body's structural and functional components. Anabolic reactions require energy, which is supplied by the catabolic reactions of the body. Fats also participate in the body's anabolism. For instance, fats can be built into the phospholipids that form the plasma membrane, and they are also part of the steroid hormones.

When the body needs energy, the glycogen stored in the liver is broken down into glucose and released into the bloodstream to be transported to cells, where it will be catabolized. This process, called glycogenolysis, usually occurs between meals.

NUTRIENTS

Nutrients are chemical substances in food that provide energy, form new body components, or assist in the functioning of various body processes. There are six principal classes of nutrients—carbohydrates, lipids (fats), proteins, water, minerals, and vitamins. Carbohydrates, lipids, and proteins are digested by enzymes in the gastrointestinal tract. The end products of digestion that ultimately reach body cells are different forms of sugar, amino acids, and fatty acids. Some nutrients are used to synthesize new structural molecules in cells, or to synthesize new regulatory molecules, such as enzymes and hormones, but most nutrients are used to produce energy to sustain life processes, including acting as active transport, DNA replication, synthesis of proteins and other molecules, muscle contraction, and nerve-impulse conduction.

Some minerals and many vitamins are integral to the enzyme systems. They catalyze the reactions of the macronutrients—carbohydrates, lipids, and proteins—breaking them down chemically so they can become useful to the body. Even the most well-balanced diet may not sufficiently replenish all the vitamins, minerals, and foodstuffs used up by athletes in training and competition, so certain supplements must be taken, and at specific times, in order to maximize their effect on the body. This is usually done during the restorative phase following exercise.

Many people are very limited in their beliefs and prejudices regarding nutritional practices. And athletes are continually looking for special foods and diets that will help improve their performance. Unfortunately, many athletes are not knowledgeable about nutrition, and proper supplementation is often necessary to assure a balanced level of nutrition. Nutritional supplements should be taken for increased work capacity and recovery time, not solely to compensate for used energy or nutrient-poor meals. Any effort rapidly uses up vitamins and minerals, and stress destroys these vital chemicals.

Carbohydrates

These macronutrients are your primary source of instant available energy for external and internal activity. There are basically two types of carbohydrates, simple (fast) and complex (slow). Simple carbohydrates are sugars, starches, and white-flour products. Complex carbohydrates are fruits, seeds, vegetables (preferably green), and whole grains and their products. Sugars and starches are converted in the digestive system into blood sugar (glucose), then stored in the brain, liver, and muscle. How fast the supply of energy depletes depends on the source.

Refined carbohydrates release and deplete quickly, while more complex carbohydrates convert to glucose, and are used at a slower rate. Your ability to train effectively is hampered by sugar withdrawal, where your supply of sugar simply runs out and disorientation and fatigue set in. Your body needs to store as much glycogen (stored glucose) as possible in order to enhance performance, calm the body, and free the mind. The best way to do this is to make sure you have plenty of complex carbohydrates stored in the liver. To do this, you must eat three hours prior to any training session (this is known as carb loading). In addition, have a simple carbohydrate, a sugary drink, for example, on hand throughout your workout. It is important to take in large amounts of fluids while you're training, for every gram of water holds 1 gram of carbohydrates in the muscle. When you sweat out the water, you lose the ability to hold the glycogen in the muscle, thus depleting energy faster than necessary.

The Fate of Carbohydrates

Since glucose is the body's preferred source of energy, the fate of absorbed glucose depends on the energy needs of the body's cells. If they require immediate energy, the glucose is oxidized by them. The glucose not needed for immediate use is handled in several ways. First, the liver can convert excess glucose to glycogen. Second, if the storage areas for glycogen are filled up, the liver cells can transform the glucose to fat that can be stored in adipose tissue. Later, when the cells need more energy, the glycogen and fat can be converted back to glucose, which is released into the bloodstream so it can be transported to cells for oxidation. Without the inhibiting effects of fats or roughage, the stomach empties its contents quickly, and the carbohydrates are digested simultaneously.

During the process of digestion, polysaccharides and disaccharides are hydrolyzed to become monosaccharides—glucose, galactose, and fructose.

They are then carried to the liver, where fructose and galactose are converted to glucose (sugar). The liver is the only organ that has the enzymes necessary for this conversion. Thus, the story of carbohydrate metabolism is really the story of glucose metabolism and the liver.

If glucose is not needed immediately for energy, it is combined with many other molecules of glucose to form glycogen. This process, stimulated by insulin from the pancreas, is called glycogenesis. The body can store about 500 grams of glycogen in the liver and skeletal muscle cells (the latter store about 80 percent of the glycogen).

Lipids (Fats)

Secondly, there is fat. In general, people don't consider fats an important macronutrient in their diet. Fats have gotten much bad press, but they do serve a purpose and have a good side. Fats work with vitamins to assure their absorption. They are a secondary form of energy and help with the creation and performance of hormones.

There are basically three kinds of fats: unsaturated, hydrogenated, and saturated. Unsaturated fats are the good fats. They contain the essential fatty acids necessary for growth and the prevention of heart disease. Hydrogenated fats are not good. They are made solid by the addition of the chemical hydrogen and act in destructive ways. Read labels and avoid products made with hydrogenated fats, also called trans-fatty acids. Saturated fats are found in such animal products as butter, lard, and fatty meats. They contain an unusual number of carbon links within the fatty acids, which makes them difficult to digest. They don't burn well, and they are easily stored. Oxidized fatty acids and cholesterol lead to cardiovascular disease. This happens simply because the good cholesterol-shaking antioxidants are not present in the bloodstream due to poor food choices. Such poor nutrient intake allows oxygen to attack fat and cause damage to cells. This is certainly something you can prevent. A good antioxidant food supplement goes a long way toward preventing cellular damage. A good health food store will supply many good antioxidant products, such as beta-carotene and vitamins C and E. (*See* Table 16.2 on page 227 for a listing of recommended antioxidants.)

Fat (Lipid) Metabolism

Lipids, such as fatty acids, may oxidize to produce energy (ATP). Each gram of fat produces about 9 calories. If the body has no immediate need to utilize fats, they are stored in the skin as adipose tissue (fat depots), in the liver and throughout the body.

The major function of adipose tissue is to provide storage for fats until they are needed for energy in other parts of the body. It also insulates and protects. About 50 percent of stored fat is deposited in subcutaneous tissue, and 5 to 8 percent between the muscles. Fats are renewed about once every two to three weeks, so the fat stored in your adipose tissue today is not the same fat that was there last month. Fat is continually released from storage, transported, and redeposited back into adipose-tissue cells.

The body can store much more fat than it can glycogen. Moreover, the energy yield of fats is more than twice that of carbohydrates. Fats are the body's second favorite source of energy, but before fat molecules can be metabolized as an energy source, they must first be released from fat depots by processes that are stimulated by growth hormone (GH).

Liver cells burn fat, sugar, and protein through a process called lipo-genesis. When a greater amount of carbohydrates enters the body than is required for energy, or to be stored as glycogen, the carbohydrates will be synthesized into fats in a process enhanced by insulin. This holds true for amino acids as well. When people have more proteins in their diet than can be utilized, much of the excess protein is converted to, and stored as, fats.

Protein

Protein is a builder. Its primary goal is to produce building blocks for the body, primarily muscles, hormones, and enzymes. Protein itself is made up of its own building blocks called amino acids. There are twenty-one amino acids, eight of which are considered essential because they can be used by the body to make the other thirteen. A protein food is considered complete if it contains these eight essential amino acids, and incomplete if it is missing any one of the eight that is not made up for in a complementary food (rice and beans, for example), thus rendering it useless. When someone con-stantly eats a diet with less than these eight essential amino acids, he or she will go into a protein deficit that will cause low energy, mental and emo-tional problems, and weakness. The body will become more receptive to infection and have a difficult time recovering from illness. Muscles and bones will constantly be sore, and wounds will heal slowly. Foods such as beans, grains, or lentils that are not combined to provide all eight amino acids are essentially ineffective because they are all incomplete proteins.

Such foods as dairy products, fish, and meats are complete proteins and perform all the tasks assigned to them.

Another factor in protein consumption is the time you eat. This is critical. Generally, protein should *not* be eaten before training or exercise because it is a dense molecule and hard to digest. Blood is required for digestion, and the blood that would ordinarily contribute to performance will be trapped in the digestive system and directed away from the muscle, which will result in the denial of essential nutrients and oxygen to the muscle.

Tests have shown that the optimum time to consume protein is about an hour after exercise, and anywhere between one and two hours before bedtime. For healing and building, protein works best with human growth hormone, which is excreted during mid-sleep. The timing is mutually perfect for both, as it takes approximately four hours to digest protein, as well as to release human growth hormone.

It is advisable to eat carbohydrates two hours prior to exercising, and also immediately after because those carbohydrates will have a protein-sparing effect on the muscle. This means they will be burned as fuel first, instead of the protein, thus sparing the protein for building, healing, and at the same time raising the body's metabolism.

As stress increases, protein needs increase. Mental stress, especially, increases the need for protein. My daily recommendation is 1 gram of protein per pound of body weight, and approximately 1.42 grams during stressful times.

Make sure you eat your protein alone. As far back as biblical times, eating protein separately from carbohydrates was the law. Even then, they knew that the process of digestion for these two types of food together was not optimum. The digestive system was just not built efficiently enough to handle the processing and absorption of protein and carbohydrates at the same time.

The Fate of Proteins

Proteins enter body cells by active transport. This process is stimulated by growth hormone and insulin. Almost immediately after entrance, they are synthesized into amino acids. The body uses very little protein for energy, as long as it ingests or stores sufficient amounts of carbohydrates and fats. Each gram of protein produces about 4 calories. Most proteins function as enzymes, and are involved in transportation, serving as antibodies, clotting chemicals, and hormones in muscle cells. Several proteins serve as structural components of the body.

Protein Metabolism

During the process of digestion, proteins are broken down into their con-stituent amino acids. The amino acids are then absorbed by the blood capil-laries through the villi, and transported to the liver via the hepatic portal vein for amino acid remodelling. Since amino acids contain nitrogen, the major site of nitrogen metabolism is the liver.

Protein Catabolism

A certain amount of protein catabolism occurs in the body each day. Amino acids are extracted from worn-out cells and broken down, making new pro-teins. If other energy sources are used up, the liver can convert protein to fat or glucose (sugar), or oxidize it to carbon dioxide and water.

Protein Anabolism

Protein anabolism involves the formation of new proteins. Protein synthesis is stimulated by growth hormone, thyroxin, and insulin. The proteins are the primary constituents of antibodies, clotting chemicals, enzymes, hor-mones, structural components of cells, and so forth. Because proteins are a primary ingredient of most cell structures, high-protein diets are essential during exercise.

When your liver runs low on glycogen and you do not eat, your body starts catabolizing proteins. Unless you are starving, however, large-scale fat and protein catabolism does not occur. Both fat molecules and protein molecules may be converted in the liver to glucose. Low-calorie diets insuf-ficient to energy needs can bring about this catabolizing or wasting away.

Water and Its Dietary Importance

Water is by far the largest single constituent of the body, making up 45 to 80 percent of total body weight. The major source of water is ingested liquids and foods. A secondary source is called metabolic water that results from the body breaking down chemical bonds.

To maintain a fluid balance, the body has several ways to rid the body of waste water. The primary route of fluid output is through the kidneys, and other routes are through the gastrointestinal tract, the lungs, and the skin. It is important to maintain adequate fluid levels. Regulating your fluid intake according to thirst is an inefficient method simply because, if you're experi-encing thirst, you're already dehydrated.

Body fluids contain electrolytes, and these have three general functions in the body:

1. As essential minerals, they are necessary for survival.

2. They control the water pressure between body compartments.

3. They help maintain the acid/base balance required for normal cellular activity.

Insufficient intake of water can result in confusion, headaches, hypertension, and muscle weakness. A 10 percent reduction of water in your body can make you sick. A loss of 20 percent can mean death.

This amazing substance is involved in every bodily function known to man. A reduction in water means more concentrated blood. Thicker blood is more susceptible to clotting, less able to deliver oxygen to your brain and muscles, and less capable of transporting substances to and from your various tissues.

Temperature regulation is also controlled by water. Plus, it is responsible for the actions involved in energy production, as well as the lubrication of joints.

As an athlete, water helps you recover from your workouts, aids in the fat-based fueling of muscles, and provides crucial water storage inside your cells. When you become dehydrated, all these functions are diminished and your performance levels decline. A reduction in water can result in a 20 to 30 percent drop in physical performance. Again, don't wait until you're thirsty to drink water. By the time your body reaches that point, you are already deficient in this fluid.

The importance of water is unquestionable, especially for an athlete. As the major substance in the human body, water is essential to healthy and qualitative athletic performance. Drink from six to eight full glasses of water a day. But don't overdo it. Too much of anything can have adverse effects. This includes water. Too much water can dilute potassium levels, raising your risk of stroke. Also, here at the Atomic Institute in Farmingdale, New York, we urge clients not to drink fluoride water. Why? Because fluoride makes your body absorb aluminum, which goes directly to your brain, resulting in memory loss and other brain disorders.

Minerals

Minerals are not made by living systems. They originate in the earth and are

Dairy Products

A range of foods fall under the dairy category. Besides milk, there are cheeses, yogurt, and all sorts of creams. These creams are extremely complex, usually containing all the macronutrients (fats, proteins, and carbohydrates) together. These deadly combinations will cancel each other out, and slow down the absorption of everything else in the digestive system. Some cheeses can take as long as eight hours to be fully digested and absorbed. That's a lot of time and energy being used up. Milk and milk products often contain large amounts of hormones, antidepressants, and antibiotics, and there is some evidence they may even be sexually suppressive. Eggs are in the same category as milk, with one small exception—eggs contain a more suitable and usable protein than milk. Dairy products, overall, do not provide optimal sources of protein.

obtained from the soil by plants. Most of the minerals in the diet come directly from plants or indirectly from animal sources. Some minerals are also available through water supplies, though this varies according to geographic location. Similarly, the minerals obtained from plants depends on the soil of the particular geographic location.

Until recently, vitamins were thought to be more important to athletic performance than minerals, but vast research has shown that minerals play a highly significant role in various bodily functions and are essential to physical movement. A deficiency in any mineral can be disastrous to peak performance and health. Minerals are frequently lacking in most diets, and inadequate levels of them can result in fatigue, injury, and weakness. Since the stresses associated with sport activities promote the loss of various minerals, it becomes even more important to increase your mineral intake.

Vitamins

Everyone needs vitamins. It is best to obtain vitamins through the diet, but a vitamin supplement is also important, particularly for the athlete. However, it's important to make certain your supplements are in the form of phytonutrient complexes, which are combinations of all the nutrients found in nature, or you may be ingesting things you don't want.

Here's a little information you need to know about vitamin supplements. The companies that manufacture them use a process in which they fractionate (split) a food into its separate components. The new substances are then recombined into a pill or powder and sold to you under the pretense that they're natural. So, even if these vitamins started out as whole foods, they're anything but by the time they reach you. If you isolate a nutrient, by definition you've created a chemical, which is only a part of the whole food it came from. The human body utilizes nutrients in conjunction, or synergistically, with one another, and the only complete and body-friendly compounds are the phytonutrient complexes. Taking high dosages of fractionized supplements, or taking synthetic compounds, can result in impaired body functions.

It has been reported that store-bought supplements, which are easy and inexpensive to manufacture, can lack the digestive quality necessary for absorption and can, in some instances, be manufactured from sewage sludge (in the case of vitamin B_{12}), irradiated oil (vitamin D), or laboratory byproducts (vitamin E). Phytonutrient complexes, on the other hand, use a time-consuming process that assures their quality, so the next time you're looking for a vitamin, be very aware of what you're buying.

In any case, supplements are important to ensure that your body has the nutrients it needs. This is particularly true for athletes. A high level of activity makes it even more critical to replenish the nutrients being used. If you want to be a successful athlete, you need to provide your body with everything it needs. Each vitamin has a specific responsibility, so it's probably wise to take a moderate dosage multivitamin and mineral supplement at

Phytochemicals (Phytonutrients)

Phytochemicals are produced by plants. New research is consistently discovering how truly essential these nutrients are. While there is plenty of evidence to support the health benefits of diets rich in fruit, vegetables, whole grains, legumes, and nuts, data on the specific nutrients or phytochemicals that contribute to these benefits is only beginning to become available. Due to the fact that plant-based foods are complex mixtures of bioactive compounds, information about the individual phytochemicals is linked to information on the health effects of the foods that contain those phytochemicals.

least once a day. Caution must be taken, however, when fat-soluble vitamins (A, D, E, and K) are consumed in large quantities because of the possibility of toxicity stemming from bodily storage of these vitamins. (*See* Tables 16.1–16.3 for listings of recommended vitamins and minerals, antioxidants, and herbs and super foods.)

TABLE 16.1. RECOMMENDED VITAMINS AND MINERALS

Vitamins and Minerals	What They Support
Biotin	Energy, hair, and skin
Boron (chelate)	Bones and muscles
Calcium (carbonate, citrate, malate, ascorbate)	Bones, gums, and teeth
Choline (bitartrate)	Brain and liver
Chromium (polynicotinate)	Blood sugar and energy
Copper (chelate)	Bones and joints
Folic acid	Heart and brain
Hesperidin (citrus peel)	Immune system and joints
Inositol	Hair and nerves
Iodine	Energy and immunity
Lemon bioflavonoid complex	Blood vessels and bruising
Magnesium (oxide, aspartate, ascorbate)	Blood pressure
Manganese (aspartate, ascorbate)	Blood sugar and energy
Molybdenum (chelate)	Energy and gums
N-acetyl cysteine (NAC)	Immune system
Niacin (niacinamide niacin)	Cholesterol and heart
Pantothenic acid (calcium pantothenate)	Energy
Para-aminobenzoic acid (PABA)	Blood and intestines
Potassium	Energy and water balance
Quercetin (as dihydrate)	Heart
Rutin (buckwheat)	Immune system and joints
Selenium (chelate)	Immune system
Silica (horsetail extract, silicon dioxide)	Arteries, joints, and nails
Trace minerals	Energy and metabolism
Vanadium (chelate)	Bones and cholesterol
Vitamin A (retinyl palmitate)	Eyes

Vitamins and Minerals	What They Support
Vitamin B_1 (thiamine) (mononitrate)	Energy
Vitamin B_2 (riboflavin)	Cell development and eyes
Vitamin B_6 (pyridoxine HCL, pyridoxal-5-phosphate)	Brain, heart, and immunity
Vitamin B_{12} (cyanocobalamin)	Blood and nerves
Vitamin C (ascorbic acid, calcium ascorbate, manganese ascorbate)	Immune system
Vitamin D (cholecalciferol)	Bones
Vitamin K (phytonadione)	Blood and bones
Zinc (chelate)	Immunity and prostate

TABLE 16.2. RECOMMENDED ANTIOXIDANTS

Antioxidants	What They Support
Alpha-lipoic acid	Immune system
Coenzyme Q_{10} (ubiquinone)	Energy and heart
Lutein (as lutein esters from marigolds)	Eyes and immune system
Lycopene (tomatoes)	Immune system and prostate
Tocotrienols (rice bran oil)	Cholesterol and heart
Vitamin A (beta-carotene)	Immune system
Vitamin C (ascorbic acid, calcium ascorbate, manganese ascorbate)	Immune system
Vitamin E (d-alpha tocopherol, mixed tocopherols)	Heart and immune system

TABLE 16.3. RECOMMENDED HERBS AND SUPER FOODS

This is a list of wonderful resources to help support and maintain a healthy body.

Herbs and Super Foods	What They Support
Amylase	Absorption and digestion
Astragalus (root)	Immune system
Bee pollen	Immune system
Betaine hydrochloride (HCL)	Absorption of nutrients
Cellulose	Absorption and digestion

Herbs and Super Foods	What They Support
Eleuthero root (and extract)	Endurance and energy
Ginger (root)	Circulation and digestion
Ginkgo biloba extract (leaf)	Brain and circulation
Green tea extract (leaf)	Cholesterol and immunity
Gymnema sylvestre (leaf)	Blood sugar
L-carnitine (tartarate)	Energy and heart
Lipase	Absorption and digestion, emulsifies fat
L-taurine	Brain
Maltase	Absorption and digestion
Ox bile	Absorption of nutrients
Panax ginseng root (and extract)	Immune system and stress
Pancreatin (porcine)	Transportation of nutrients
Protease	Absorption and digestion, emulsifies fat
Royal jelly	Immune system and normal cholesterol
Spirulina (algae)	Immune system
Turmeric (root)	Immune system and liver

A RESOURCE LIST: RICH NUTRIENTS AND THEIR SOURCES

Items marked with an asterisk (*) may contain substances that could interact negatively with certain medications. If you are taking drugs, consult a healthcare professional before adding any supplements to your diet.

Vitamin A (Carotene) (Fat-Soluble)

Alfalfa*
Butter
Carrots
Fish-liver oils*

Liver*
Vegetables, dark green
Vegetables, yellow and orange

Vitamin B (All B Vitamins Are Water-Soluble)

Vitamin B Complex

Brewer's yeast*
Desiccated liver and liver*

Wheat germ*

Vitamin B₁ (Thiamine)

Green peas
Lean ham and pork
Luncheon meats
Muscle meats

Nuts
Oranges
Sausages
Whole-grain products

Vitamin B₂ (Riboflavin)

Cottage cheese, milk, and whey
Dried beans and peas
Egg whites
Fish

Muscle meats and tongue
Oysters
Whole-grain products

Vitamin B₆ (Pyridoxine)

Eggs
Fresh fruits and vegetables
Molasses*
Muscle meats

Nuts and seeds
Soybean products
Unpolished rice
Whole-grain products

Vitamin B₁₂ (Cyanocobalamin)

Cheese
Egg yolk
Kelp

Liver*
Whole milk

Vitamin B₁₅ (Pangamic Acid)

Brown rice
Liver*
Pumpkin seeds

Rice bran
Sesame seeds
Sunflower seeds

Biotin

Cauliflower
Egg yolk
Muscle meats
Organ meats*
Salmon

Sardines
Soybean products
Unpolished rice
Whole-grain products

Choline

Beans and peas
Egg yolks and milk
Kidneys and liver*
Muscle meats

Nuts
Soybean products
Spinach

Folic Acid (Folacin)

Desiccated liver and liver*   Legumes
Green leafy vegetables   Muscle meats

Inositol

Beef brains and heart   Dried beans and peas
Blackstrap molasses*   Fruits and raisins
Cabbage   Peanuts

Niacin (Nicotinic Acid)

Fish   Peanut butter
Liver*   Poultry
Muscle meats   Whole-grain products

PABA (Para-Aminobenzoic Acid)

Eggs   Molasses*
Liver*   Rice bran
Milk

Pantothenic Acid

Cheese   Milk
Egg yolks   Peanuts
Liver*   Whole-grain products

Vitamin C (Ascorbic Acid) (Water-Soluble)

Acerola (Puerto-Rican cherry)   Rose hips
Citrus fruits   Strawberries
Green leafy vegetables   Tomatoes
Green peppers

Vitamin D (Fat-Soluble)

Butter   Liver*
Eggs   Milk (fortified)
Fish liver oil*   Saltwater fish

Vitamin E (Fat-Soluble)

Green leafy vegetables   Nuts
Milk and eggs   Sunflower seeds

Legumes
Liver

Vegetable oils
Wheat germ and wheat germ oil

Vitamin F (Unsaturated Fatty Acids)

Fish liver oil*
Golden vegetable oils (corn,
   safflower, soy)

Nuts
Salad dressings
Sunflower seeds

Vitamin K (Menadione K) (Fat-Soluble)

Alfalfa*
Cabbage
Egg yolks
Fish liver oil*
Green leafy vegetables

Liver*
Molasses*
Soybean products
Spinach

Vitamin P (Riboflavonoids, Rutin) (Water-Soluble)

Grapes
Plums
Prunes

Rose hips
White segments of citrus fruits

Minerals

Calcium

Bone meal
Cheese
Fish

Green leafy vegetables
Milk
Yogurt

Chlorine

Green Leafy vegetables
Muscle meats
Organ meats*

Rye flour
Salt
Seaweed (dulse, kelp)

Iodine

Dried beans
Iodized salt
Mushrooms

Seafood
Seaweed (dulse, kelp)

Iron

Brewer's yeast*
Desiccated liver*
Dried fruits

Muscle and organ meats*
Oysters
Wheat germ

Magnesium

Figs
Kelp
Nuts
Pumpkin and sunflower seeds

Soybean products
Wheat germ
Whole-grain products

Manganese

Beets
Dried beans and peas
Egg yolks

Green leafy vegetables
Sunflower seeds
Whole-grain products

Phosphorus

Bone meal
Dried beans and peas
Eggs
Meat

Nuts
Sunflower seeds
Whole-grain products

Potassium

Citrus fruits
Figs
Fish
Green peppers
Meat

Mint leaves
*Molasses
Watercress
Whole-grain products

Sodium

Beets
carrots
Green leafy vegetables
Kelp

Seafood
Sea salt
Table salt

Trace Minerals

Copper

Dried beans and peas
Egg yolks
Liver*

Prunes
Shrimp
Whole-grain products

Fluorine

Bone meal
Mineral water
Ocean fish

Rose hips
Sea salt
Seaweed

Vanadium and Other Trace Minerals

Bone meal
Brewer's yeast*
Green leafy vegetables
Kelp
Mineral water

Rose hips
Saltwater fish
Sea salt
Whole-grain products

Zinc

Eggs
Fish
Liver*
Milk

Nuts
Poultry
Sunflower seeds
Wheat germ

Protein and Amino Acids

Brewer's yeast*
Cheese
Dried beans and peas
Fish
Eggs

Milk
Muscle and organ meats*
Sesame seeds
Soybean products
Wheat germ

Lecithin (Fatty Substances)

Cold-pressed oils
Egg yolks
Granulated lecithin supplement

Soybeans
Sunflower seeds
Whole-grain products

DID YOU KNOW?
Helpful Hints and Tidbits for Weight Loss and Dieting

1. If you are constantly fatigued, experience digestive problems, and have a bloated stomach regardless of how much fat or weight you have lost, you could have a sensitivity to wheat and wheat products. The gluten in wheat can cause inflammation of the stomach and digestive tract, keeping the stomach and intestine artificially bloated and making a lot of people look ten to twenty pounds heavier than they really are. They look pushed out because the air pressure inside their bodies becomes stronger than their stomach muscles, and all the sit-ups and abdominal classes in the world will not flatten a bloated stomach. If this is you, avoid wheat at all costs. Why look overweight if you don't have to?

2. I have discovered a key reason why diets ultimately fail and how you can keep this from happening: Most diets don't work because they are the wrong diets, at the wrong time, for the wrong people. After you have discovered the right way to eat for your body's particular requirements (as discussed), there are several additional elements to consider that will further increase your diet's effectiveness. The first is called *the amino connection*, specifically the amino acid tryptophan. Tryptophan is the nutrient that causes people to feel full, content, and satisfied at the end of a meal. Tryptophan eliminates that deprived feeling that causes you to cheat on your diet. Tryptophan as a supplement can be hard to find, but there's another supplement, *Griffonia simplicifolia*, that is even more effective than tryptophan and ten times more potent. Use it and be energized and full of life—you'll feel and look great.

3. I have already discussed how excess blood sugar makes you fat. When a simple carbohydrate or sugar releases into the bloodstream, the excess sugar in the blood is quickly absorbed and stored as fat. A little secret that bodybuilders have used with great success is to take a natural, high-fiber product called konjac. Konjac slows down and evens out the release of food energy when you take it before a meal. Its effects are miraculous. A mere gram of konjac provides the same

amount of fiber as twelve apples or a whole bag of prunes. Ask your health food expert about it and get started.

4. I have stressed the fact that you should never consume fruit with a meal. Fruit should be consumed separately, as a meal of its own. However, there does seem to be an exception to this rule. After a three-group study, researchers at the Scripps Clinic in San Diego concluded that those who ate grapefruit with each meal lost an average of 3.6 pounds, three times more than those who did not. Researchers believe that grapefruit contains certain biochemicals with properties that assist in the management of insulin (insulin spikes are among the chief causes of excess body fat).

5. Can't get rid of that trunk-area body fat? Recently, the National Institutes of Health published a study that examined the benefits of calcium on lower waist and trunk-area body fat. They found evidence that individuals with the highest levels of calcium had the greatest instances of weight loss. Those with low calcium levels tended to have elevated body weight.

6. Most everyone, especially dieters, has used artificial sweeteners in place of sugar. One of the best sugar substitutes I have found is stevia, a natural product extracted from *Stevia rebaudiana*, a small plant native to Paraguay and Brazil. This herb helps suppress the glucose response that is an absolute in fat loss according to the Food and Drug Administration.

7. Eating fat will not make you fat. Scientists have proved this. They have discovered that if the fat you're eating contains, or is supplemented with, conjugated linoleic acid (CLA), it has a slimming effect on the body. Thanks to new research, it is now known that CLA's job is to make sure fats are converted into muscle and energy. Without CLA, fats are simply stored.

8. Flax fights fat. In fact, next to CLA, nothing transforms the human body into a fat-burning machine better than flaxseed oil. Start with 3 tablespoons of flax-oil supplement daily. Continue until you've achieved your desired weight loss, then cut back to 1 teaspoon a day.

9. Want to spike your metabolism? Try eating mustard before your workout. I'm talking about the hot, spicy variety found in Asian markets

or gourmet food stores. A professor of the Oxford Polytechnic Institute found that a teaspoon of Asian mustard can temporarily speed up your metabolism as much as 20 to 25 percent for several hours.

10. Studies in Switzerland demonstrated that when green-tea capsules were taken with a meal, the participants burned an additional 80 calories, most of them from fat. A good dosage of green tea would be 90–100 milligrams taken with each meal.

11. Popeye wasn't too far off with his spinach. Researchers at the University of Texas found that spinach, rich in vitamins C and E, has the ability to rev up the metabolism and burn fat. Also, due to the fact that it's rich in beta-carotene, spinach has a bounty of nutrients and only a few calories.

12. Estrogen dominance is a condition seldom talked about. Overweight or overstressed men and women are at particular risk. Fatty tissue increases the conversion of testosterone to estrogen. This provokes further weight gain and fatty tissue. DIM (di-indolemethane) is a natural plant nutrient found in some vegetables. It can greatly control and improve estrogen metabolism, aiding in the body's ability to metabolize fat. You can find DIM at any good health food store.

13. Having joint problems after a workout? Glucosamine and chondroitin sulfates are good, and you should use them to help with inflammation and regeneration of cartilage. If you find, however, that these sulfates are failing you at some level, try this remedy: Mix a tablespoon of soy powder with half an avocado. Make a paste out of it and eat it after your workout. This little trick can help you build strong, thicker cartilage and give you greater mobility.

14. Want to live longer and feel stronger? Then tell those exercise fanatics to take a walk. Yes, walking is better than running, especially marathon running. Statistics show that marathon runners die suddenly nearly 200 times more often than those who walk. Conclusion: A lot of long, drawn-out exercise—no good. A lot of short-duration exercise—excellent.

15. The amino acid, L-arginine, is very popular in muscle-building circles due to the fact that it is a growth-hormone releaser. Growth hormone promotes fat burning and muscle building. Certain foods

contain L-arginine, including pork, which is one of the best sources of this amino acid. Twelve to 16 ounces of pork provide almost 5 grams of L-arginine.

16. Want to increase your recovery ability after a good workout or stressful day? Researchers at Louisville Medical School found a compound called glutathione. It's a tripeptide composed of three amino acids. Its major functions are regulating protein and cell growth, maintaining the strength and integrity of the cell, and detoxification. You can also help your muscles grow and recover more easily by consuming cruciferous vegetables, such as broccoli (not the stem) and Brussels sprouts.

17. Proper pH levels are essential in building muscle and bone. The pH level measures acidity and alkalinity in substances. It is beneficial to have a slightly more alkaline pH level. Researchers have discovered that the bones serve as an acid-reducing facility for the body, another good reason to maintain strong, healthy bones. It is quite a dichotomy that researchers in Germany have discovered that, while dairy is basically good for bones, certain cheeses are not. They have found that the sharper the cheese, the more acidic it is. To counteract the effect of a high-acid diet, try using potassium bicarbonate. It has a sparing effect on muscle tissue.

18. Want to go nuts over losing weight? Research has repeatedly shown that by simply eating nuts, you can improve your fat metabolism. A good nut combination is almonds, hazelnuts, pecans, and walnuts. These nuts are nearly a perfect food, but please limit your intake to no more than 3 ounces a day. This will provide an ample amount of good fatty acids and the amino acid L-arginine. So be a nut and live longer.

19. Millions of Americans experience exhaustion and unwanted pounds. An underactive thyroid can cause this effect. To rebalance this condition, a good natural solution I have personally found useful is to take two drops of a liquid iodine product called Losol (*not* antiseptic or topical iodine), which can be found at your local health food store, along with 30 milligrams of zinc, and 100 milligrams of selenium. Good luck.

20. Are you hot to trot over fat loss? Then try eating hot pepper, or take capsaicin capsules twice a day. These will safely increase your energy levels and remove fat molecules.

21. Haven't had much personal experience with this one, but NFL players swear by it. If you're experiencing muscle cramps, eat a slice of sour pickle. They say it will help within sixty seconds. Also, to prevent those cramps in the first place, they recommend drinking 2 ounces of pickle juice before and after your workout. Give it a try.

22. You may think I've lost my mind when you read this one, but don't discount it too quickly. To relieve muscle pain and soreness, just create usable electron energy. All you need is 18 inches of PVC pipe and some fake fur. Rub the pipe against the fur several times. Then, slowly move the pipe about a half inch to an inch above the sore area of your body. Repeat rubbing the pipe with the fur and passing it over the affected area. It's simple, harmless, and it works.

23. Turn your body into a fat-burning machine. Try an ancient Ayurvedic secret to jump-start your metabolism. It's called *Garcinia cambogia*, and it's made from the dried rind of the Indian fruit garcinia. Research has shown that the active ingredient, hydroxycitrate (HCA), can effectively control appetite and maximize the utilization of carbohydrates. Lab analysis also suggests that HCA boosts metabolism and promotes the oxidation (or breakdown) of fats. HCA may even boost your mood by safely increasing the brain chemical serotonin.

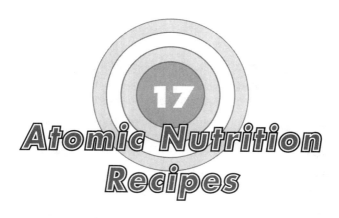

Atomic Nutrition Recipes

In this chapter I've put together a few recipes designed to provide maximum benefits to the body, recipes that really deliver the nutritional goods, Atomic style. Here you'll find not only a wonderful breakfast oatmeal to add to your repertoire, but also delicious and healthy fish, steak, pork, chicken, turkey, and vegetable dishes. And for special treats, check out the desserts at the end of the chapter. To help you choose meals appropriate to your specific diet needs, I have included nutritional information at the end of each recipe.

All nutritional information in these recipes is from the USDA National Nutrient Database for Standard Reference.

BREAKFAST

UP-THE-DOSAGE OATMEAL

This is truly a carbohydrate-day breakfast (makes a great pre-workout meal, too). Oatmeal is an excellent way to boost your metabolism and start your day with low-glycemic (slow-digesting), nutrient-dense, fiber-rich foods. The essential (good) fats in the almonds will satisfy your hunger and help keep you fueled for hours. It doesn't get much easier than this to whip up a great breakfast in just a few minutes.

YIELD: ONE SERVING

$^1/_2$ cup raw old-fashioned oats

1 tablespoon natural, unsalted almond butter

$1/2$ ounce (about 12 whole kernels) raw,
unsalted, chopped almonds

$1/4$ cup extra-fiber All-Bran cereal

Stevia sweetener to taste, optional

Cook oats as directed on package (I prefer microwave directions; it's faster).
When cooked to your liking, stir in the other ingredients and enjoy.

Variation: Natural peanut butter and peanuts can be substituted for the
almond butter and almonds.

Nutritional Information
Calories: 347

Protein: 13.50 grams

Fat: 18.20 grams

Carbohydrates: 29.15 grams (net carbohydrates;
fiber deducted from total)

Fiber: 13.70 grams

FISH

BAKED SALMON WITH BOK CHOY

*Baking salmon at a high temperature gives it a thick,
crunchy crust, while keeping it moist inside. Bok choy,
also known as Chinese cabbage, is a mild, quick-cooking
green, high in potassium, vitamin A, and vitamin C.*

YIELD: FOUR SERVINGS

2 tablespoons olive oil

2 pounds salmon fillet, cut into 4 portions

$1/2$ teaspoon salt, optional

$1/4$ teaspoon lemon pepper

$1 1/2$ pounds bok choy, cut into $1 1/2$-inch pieces

Heat oven to 475°F. Place olive oil in a skillet large enough to hold fish in a single layer. Place in oven 3 minutes. Season fish with salt and lemon pepper. Place fish flesh-side down in prepared skillet. Bake 10 minutes, turning carefully once halfway through cooking time, until just cooked through. Remove salmon from skillet and lightly cover with foil. Add bok choy to skillet. Stir to coat with pan's oil. Place in oven 1 minute, until the leaves are wilted and the stems are warmed through.

Nutritional Information (per serving)
Calories: 392.75
Protein: 36.40 grams
Fat: 25.55 grams
Carbohydrates: 2 grams (net carbohydrates; fiber deducted from total)
Fiber: 1.70 grams

CUMIN CORIANDER SWORDFISH

Cumin and coriander are the perfect partners to add great flavor to grilled swordfish. A simple green salad is all you need to complete this high-protein, low-fat meal.

YIELD: FOUR SERVINGS

1 $\frac{1}{2}$ teaspoons ground coriander seed, coarsely crushed

1 tablespoon cumin seed, coarsely crushed

$\frac{1}{2}$ teaspoon salt, optional

$\frac{1}{2}$ teaspoon fresh ground black pepper

4 fresh swordfish steaks, about 5 ounces and 1-inch thick

Preheat grill or nonstick grill pan to medium. In a small bowl, combine seasonings. Rub on fish. Cook 5–7 minutes per side, until fish is opaque in center and flakes easily with a fork.

Nutritional Information (per serving)
Calories: 175
Protein: 28.60 grams
Fat: 5.80 grams
Carbohydrates: 0 grams

LEAN & MEAN LEMON-PEPPER FLOUNDER AND SPINACH

Flounder is such a delicate fish that it's hard to cook in a pan without breaking (or destroying completely) the fillet. Baking it in an aluminum foil pouch, resting atop a bed of fresh spinach is the perfect solution.
The fish stays intact and remains moist and flavorful.

YIELD: FOUR SERVINGS

4 sheets aluminum foil, at least 3 inches longer than the fillets

Cooking spray, olive-oil flavor

2 cups fresh spinach, washed and dried

2 cloves fresh garlic, chopped

1 $^1/_2$ pounds flounder fillets

Dash of salt, optional

2 teaspoons lemon pepper

Heat oven to 350°F. Spray the cooking spray in the center of each of the aluminum foil sheets. Lay $^1/_2$ cup of the spinach and $^1/_4$ of the chopped garlic in the center. Place a fillet on top. Spray fillet with cooking spray and sprinkle with salt and lemon pepper. Fold ends of foil to make a pouch. Repeat until all four pouches are filled.

Place pouches on baking sheet and bake for 10–15 minutes, or until fish flakes easily with a fork. Remove from pouches and serve. Be careful when opening pouches, as steam has accumulated inside.

Nutritional Information (per serving)
Calories: 160.50
Protein: 32.55 grams
Fat: 2.05 grams
Carbohydrates: 0.69 grams (net carbohydrates;
                          fiber deducted from total)
Fiber: 0.32 grams

BEEF

DISAGREE AND GO-FREE LONDON BROIL

*This is a treat, as red meat should not be consumed too often,
so make it on a special occasion and enjoy. A perfect side dish would
be Feel-the-Burn Roasted Asparagus (see page 252), or a simple salad of
baby greens drizzled with olive oil and vinegar. Marinating the steak
(overnight if possible) will allow the flavors to be absorbed.*

YIELD: SIX SERVINGS

1 1/2 pounds top round (leanest cut) London broil

1 tablespoon fresh chopped rosemary

4 large cloves fresh garlic, finely minced

Dash of salt, optional

Fresh ground black pepper, to taste

Nonfat cooking spray

Remove any excess fat from London broil. Combine rosemary, garlic, salt, and pepper. Coat meat with mixture. Let marinate for at least 2 hours. Spray grill with nonfat cooking spray, if cooking on stovetop, or pre-heat outdoor grill until well heated.

Grill for about 5–7 minutes on each side, depending on thickness of steak and preference. Be careful not to overcook, as this will toughen the meat. Remove from heat and let stand about 10–15 minutes before carving to serve.

Nutritional Information (per serving)
Calories: 245
Protein: 40.40 grams
Fat: 8.05 grams
Carbohydrates: 0 grams

PORK

PEC-DEC PORK TENDERLOIN

The tenderloin is a very lean cut of pork, containing fewer than 4 grams of fat, and packing almost 24 grams of muscle-building, fat-burning protein per 4-ounce (pre-cooked weight) serving. This is a quick, low-prep-time recipe—perfect for the person on the go.

YIELD: EACH 4-OUNCE PORK TENDERLOIN IS A SINGLE SERVING

Fresh pork tenderloin (trimmed of any excess fat)

Garlic, rosemary, marjoram, and thyme, chopped (fresh is always best; however, dry will suffice if you can't get fresh).

Fresh ground black pepper

Nonstick cooking spray

Trim the tenderloin of any excess fat. Chop the garlic and herbs, spread on the tenderloin, and add black pepper. Store in an airtight plastic container in the refrigerator overnight. This will add flavor and tenderize the meat. If you can't prepare the night before, let it marinate for at least a few hours before cooking. The longer it marinates, the more flavorful the meat will be.

When ready to cook, preheat oven to 375°F. Spray the rack of roasting pan with nonstick cooking spray, place tenderloin on rack and spray that, too. Roast until a meat thermometer reads 160°F when inserted at the thickest part of the tenderloin. Cooking times will vary according to weight of tenderloin. Remove from oven and let sit for about 15 minutes before slicing. Serve with a fresh spinach and baby greens salad and enjoy.

Nutritional Information (per 4-ounce pork tenderloin)
Calories: 136

Protein: 23.82 grams

Fat: 3.87 grams

Carbohydrates: 0 grams

PORK TENDERLOIN WITH ROASTED GARLIC AND SAGE

Pork tenderloin is a very lean cut of pork, having just 2.5 grams of fat per 4-ounce serving and packing 24 grams of protein. The distinctive flavors of the roasted garlic and sage are a perfect complement to this mild meat.

YIELD: FOUR SERVINGS

2 teaspoons chopped fresh sage

$1/2$ teaspoon ground cinnamon

$1/8$ teaspoon ground nutmeg

6 large garlic cloves, cut in half

$1/2$ teaspoon salt, divided, optional

Nonfat cooking spray

$1 1/2$ pounds pork tenderloin
(visible fat removed)

$1/2$ teaspoon black pepper

Chopped parsley, optional

Heat oven to 450°F. Combine sage, cinnamon, nutmeg, and garlic. Add $1/4$ teaspoon salt, mix well. Spread spice mixture on a baking sheet or shallow roasting pan coated with cooking spray. Sprinkle pork tenderloin with $1/4$ teaspoon salt and pepper, and place on top of spice mixture. Bake at 450°F for 30 minutes, or until pork is done (meat thermometer reads 160°F in the thickest part). Remove from pan and keep warm. Partially mash the spice mixture with a potato masher, and serve with pork. Sprinkle with parsley, if desired.

Nutritional Information (per serving)
Calories: 210.75

Protein: 36 grams

Fat: 5.80 grams

Carbohydrates: 1.40 grams (net carbohydrates;
fiber deducted from total)

Fiber: 0.10 grams

CHICKEN

BUFF CHICKEN WINGS

*Finger food at its best. Whip up a batch of these crispy hot wings
for a sure-fire crowd pleaser.*

YIELD: SIX SERVINGS

2 large egg whites

1 cup cider vinegar

$1/4$ cup canola oil

1 teaspoon salt

$1/2$ teaspoon pepper

$1/2$ teaspoon garlic powder

$1/4$ teaspoon celery salt

Cayenne, to taste

2 pounds chicken wings (separated at joint,
and wing tips discarded)

Heat oven to 450°F. Beat egg in a medium bowl. Add vinegar, oil, salt,
pepper, garlic powder, celery salt, and cayenne. Stir until well combined.
Dip chicken pieces into marinade and arrange on a large baking pan. Bake
30 minutes, turning and brushing with marinade several times, until wings
are crisp.

Tip: If you want to drastically reduce the fat content, remove the skin from
the chicken wings before baking. This will eliminate more than 8.5 grams
of fat per serving.

Nutritional Information (per serving)

	With Skin	*Without Skin*
Calories:	304.35 grams	241.35 grams
Protein:	21.25 grams	24.20 grams
Fat:	24.06 grams	15.5 grams
Carbohydrates:	0 grams	0 grams

Jacked-Up Chicken Breasts

Chicken breasts (skinless and fat removed) are one of the best low-fat sources of protein. This is a very simple, one-pan recipe that requires almost no prep time and can be made in advance for quick meals on the go.

YIELD: FOUR SERVINGS

4 7-ounce chicken breasts, boneless, skinless,
and all visible fat removed

Nonstick cooking spray

1 tablespoon dried oregano

1 tablespoon dried, crushed rosemary

1 tablespoon lemon pepper

4 cups chopped or whole frozen spinach

2 ounces shredded or finely chopped 75% fat-free cheddar cheese

Dash of salt, optional

Heat oven to 375°F. Place chicken (one breast at a time) in a plastic freezer bag, pound lightly with a mallet. Spray a shallow baking pan with the nonstick spray, place chicken in pan, and spray lightly with the cooking spray. Sprinkle with the herbs, salt, and lemon pepper, and place in oven.

Take spinach out and let sit while chicken is cooking. Cook chicken for about 20–25 minutes, then add the frozen spinach. Just pour it on top of the chicken and cover with aluminum foil for about 10–15 minutes, or until the spinach is cooked. It is recommended to cook the chicken until a meat thermometer (inserted into the thickest part of the breast) reads 160°F.

Remove from oven, sprinkle cheese on top, and let stand for about 15 minutes (loosely covered) before serving.

Nutritional Information (per serving)

Calories: 235

Protein: 50 grams

Fat: 4.50 grams

Carbohydrates: 2 grams (net carbohydrates;
fiber deducted from total)

Fiber: 4.80 grams

HEEP IT COMIN' CORIANDER CHICHEN

If you like coriander (also known as cilantro), you'll love this dish. The addition of turmeric gives it that little extra burst of flavor. If you can't find fresh snap peas, snow peas or broccoli will make fine substitutes.

YIELD: FOUR SERVINGS

$1\frac{1}{2}$ pounds chicken cutlets, or boneless,
skinless chicken breasts

$1\frac{1}{4}$ teaspoons ground coriander

$\frac{1}{2}$ teaspoon garlic powder

$\frac{1}{2}$ teaspoon salt, optional

$\frac{1}{8}$ teaspoon ground turmeric

2 tablespoons olive oil

1 pound sugar snap peas

$\frac{3}{4}$ cup chicken broth (low sodium)

$\frac{1}{4}$ cup water

$1\frac{1}{2}$ teaspoons cilantro leaves

If using chicken breasts, slice each piece in half horizontally, place chicken inside of a freezer bag, and pound lightly with a mallet to make flat, thin pieces. Combine coriander, garlic, salt, and turmeric. Pat onto chicken. Heat oil in large skillet over medium heat. Sauté chicken 3–4 minutes per side until golden and cooked through. Remove chicken to platter, lightly cover with foil.

In a separate pan, steam sugar snap peas about 3 minutes, or until crisp-tender. Meanwhile, combine broth, water, and cilantro. Add to skillet and bring to a boil. Reduce heat to simmer, cook 1 minute. Serve over chicken with sugar snap peas.

Nutritional Information (per serving)

Calories: 289.25

Protein: 42.30 grams

Fat: 9.15 grams

Carbohydrates: 4.25 grams (net carbohydrates;
fiber deducted from total)

Fiber: 3.85 grams

TURKEY

BODY-TO-DIE-FOR TERIYAKI TURKEY CUTLETS

Served on a bed of green beans, these teriyaki turkey cutlets make a delicious and quick weeknight meal.

YIELD: FOUR SERVINGS

2 tablespoons low-sodium soy sauce

2 teaspoons grated fresh ginger root

2 cloves garlic, pushed through a press

1 packet stevia (sugar substitute)

1 1/2 pounds turkey breast cutlets

2 tablespoons canola oil, divided

2 cups frozen French-cut string beans, thawed

1 teaspoon sesame oil, divided

1 tablespoon toasted sesame seeds

Mix soy sauce, ginger, garlic, and stevia in a large bowl. Add turkey cutlets and turn to coat. Marinate in refrigerator at least 1 hour. Heat 1 tablespoon canola oil over medium-high heat in large nonstick skillet. Stir-fry vegetables until hot; toss with 1 teaspoon sesame oil. Transfer to a platter and keep warm.

Wipe out skillet. Heat remaining canola oil in skillet. Remove turkey cutlets from marinade. Discard marinade. Cook turkey cutlets 2–3 minutes per side until cooked through. Drizzle with remaining sesame oil. Serve over vegetables. Sprinkle with sesame seeds.

Nutritional Information (per serving)

Calories: 317

Protein: 44.15 grams

Fat: 11.85 grams

Carbohydrates: 4.6 grams (net carbohydrates; fiber deducted from total)

Fiber: 2.5 grams

TIP-TOP TURKEY BURGERS

A fresh turkey breast contains just one little gram of fat per 4-ounce serving, but an amazing 28 grams of protein. I use equal amounts of ground turkey breast and ground dark turkey meat to add a little more fat and flavor to these burgers. Make in advance and keep handy in the fridge to grab for a quick high-protein snack.

YIELD: TWELVE 4-OUNCE BURGERS

1$\frac{1}{2}$ pounds ground turkey breast

1$\frac{1}{2}$ pounds ground dark turkey meat

1 tablespoon dried basil

1 tablespoon chopped fresh rosemary

1 tablespoon lemon pepper

1 teaspoon garlic powder

Dash of salt, optional

Nonfat cooking spray

Combine all the ingredients in a large bowl, mix together well. Form patties, approximately 4 ounces each. Spray a large skillet with the cooking spray and heat over medium heat. Cook burgers until juices run clear, spraying lightly with cooking spray and turning two or three times to keep moist and browning evenly.

Nutritional Information (per 4-ounce burger)

Calories: 141

Protein: 24.50 grams

Fat: 4.50 grams

Carbohydrates: 0 grams

TRIPLE CROWN HERB-AND-DIJON-MUSTARD TURKEY BREAST

In this simple, yet delicious, recipe, a coating of Dijon-mustard and herbs keeps the turkey breast plump and tender.

YIELD: APPROXIMATELY SEVEN 4-OUNCE SERVINGS

Chopped fresh Italian parsley, about $1/4$ cup

1 teaspoon crushed dried sage leaves

1 teaspoon dried thyme

4–5 large fresh garlic cloves, finely minced

Dash of salt, optional

Dash of fresh ground black pepper

2 tablespoons olive oil

3 tablespoons Dijon mustard

2 tablespoons balsamic vinegar

1 boneless, skinless turkey breast (about 2 pounds)

Heat oven to 375°F. In a small bowl combine all the herbs, garlic, salt, pepper, olive oil, Dijon mustard, and balsamic vinegar to create a paste. Place turkey on a rack in a roasting pan. Brush the herb/mustard paste over top and sides of turkey. Follow directions for cooking times that are included with most turkey breasts. It is recommended to cook until a meat thermometer (inserted in the thickest part of the breast) reads 160°F. Let turkey stand 10–15 minutes before carving into slices.

Variation: The herb/mustard paste can also be used on chicken breasts, pork tenderloins, or pot roasts.

Nutritional Information (per serving)

Calories: 197

Protein: 43.57 grams

Fat: 4.95 grams

Carbohydrates: 1.25 grams (net carbohydrates;
fiber deducted from total)

Fiber: 4.0 grams

VEGETABLES

FEEL-THE-BURN ROASTED ASPARAGUS

Roasting brings out the natural sweetness in most vegetables and intensifies their flavor. Asian mustard adds a little fire and some fat-burning properties to an already healthful dish.

YIELD: FOUR SERVINGS

1 1/2 pounds slender asparagus
with tough ends snapped off

Nonfat cooking spray
(olive-oil flavor preferred)

1 teaspoon salt, optional

1/2 teaspoon black pepper

1 teaspoon Asian mustard

Heat oven to 400°F. Line a baking sheet with aluminum foil. Rinse asparagus, lightly pat dry. Spread asparagus out in pan. Spray with nonfat cooking spray and sprinkle with salt, pepper, and Asian mustard. Mix with your hands to distribute seasoning. Pat into a single layer. Bake until asparagus stalks are tender and lightly crisped, about 15 minutes. Shake pan once or twice during baking time.

Nutritional Information (per serving)
Calories: 35
Protein: 3.75 grams
Fat: 0.25 grams
Carbohydrates: 3 grams (net carbohydrates;
                    fiber deducted from total)
Fiber: 3.5 grams

SIMPLY THE BEST SAUTÉED GREENS

You can use a variety of greens, such as Swiss chard, collards, kale, mustard, or turnips, in this flavorful side dish. We're adding Asian mustard to this recipe to spice it up a bit and gain that fat-burning advantage. Purchase whichever greens are in season and look freshest.

YIELD: SIX SERVINGS

1 bunch kale (1 pound), stems removed,
torn into 2-inch pieces

1 bunch Swiss chard (1 pound), stems removed,
torn into 2-inch pieces

2 tablespoons olive oil

1 small red bell pepper, thinly sliced

1 shallot, finely chopped

$1/2$ teaspoon salt, optional

$1/2$–1 teaspoon Asian mustard

Bring a large pot of lightly salted water to boil. Add kale and Swiss chard; cook 3 minutes. Transfer to a colander and drain well. In same pot, heat oil over medium-low heat. Add bell pepper and shallot. Cook until softened, about 5 minutes. Return greens to pot. Add salt and Asian mustard to taste. Sauté until greens are tender, about 5 minutes.

Nutritional Information (per serving)

Calories: 95

Protein: 4 grams

Fat: 5.25 grams

Carbohydrates: 3 grams (net carbohydrates;
fiber deducted from total)

Fiber: 3.5 grams

VEGETABLE BARBELLS [AKA KEBABS]

Grilling is simplified by threading vegetables on skewers. Metal skewers are preferred, as they don't require soaking and won't burn. Prepare them so everything will cook in the same amount of time—that's why I'm very specific about vegetable sizes.

YIELD: SIX SERVINGS

For the Kebabs

1 baby eggplant (4 oz), cut into twelve 1-inch cubes

$1\frac{1}{4}$ teaspoons salt, divided

1 large (7 oz) red bell pepper, cut into twelve $1\frac{1}{4}$-inch-square pieces

1 large (7 oz) yellow bell pepper, cut into twelve $1\frac{1}{4}$-inch-square pieces

1 medium (8 oz) zucchini, cut into nine $\frac{3}{4}$-inch-thick pieces

1 medium (8 oz) yellow squash, cut into nine $\frac{3}{4}$-inch-thick pieces

12 cherry or grape tomatoes

$\frac{1}{4}$ teaspoon pepper

Nonfat cooking spray (olive-oil flavor)

12 large fresh basil leaves

For the Dressing

1 tablespoon minced shallots

$\frac{1}{2}$ teaspoon salt, optional

$\frac{1}{4}$ teaspoon pepper

2 tablespoons red wine vinegar

$\frac{1}{4}$ cup extra-virgin olive oil

1 tablespoon chopped fresh basil

To make the kebabs, spread eggplant cubes in a single layer on a baking sheet lined with paper towels. Sprinkle with $\frac{3}{4}$ teaspoon of the salt, and let stand 15 minutes. Pat dry. Heat grill to medium-low. In a large bowl, toss bell peppers, zucchini, squash, and cherry tomatoes with the remaining $\frac{1}{2}$ teaspoon salt and the pepper. Let sit 1 minute, and toss again with the eggplant and spray with cooking spray until well coated.

Using six 12-inch metal skewers, or six 12-inch bamboo skewers (presoaked for 20 minutes), thread each skewer with two pieces each of red and yellow bell pepper, three pieces squash or zucchini, two cubes eggplant, and two cherry tomatoes wrapped in basil leaves. Cover with plastic wrap until grill is ready. Grill until vegetables are softened and lightly browned, 15–20 minutes, turning every 5 minutes.

To make the dressing, in a small bowl, whisk all ingredients until well combined. Cover, and set aside.

Arrange kebabs on a serving platter, and drizzle with dressing. Serve immediately.

Nutritional Information (per serving)
Calories: 140
Protein: 2 grams
Fat: 12 grams
Carbohydrates: 6 grams (net carbohydrates; fiber deducted from total)
Fiber: 3 grams

MAXED-OUT SWEET POTATO HOME FRIES

Sweet potatoes are a low-glycemic, healthier, and tastier alternative to standard white potatoes. They can be used exactly like white potatoes, so don't be afraid to experiment. Here I pair up the natural sweetness of the sweet potato with cinnamon, and the combination is just perfect.

YIELD: FOUR SERVINGS

4 medium (approximately 5 inches long) sweet potatoes
Nonfat cooking spray
Ground cinnamon (**not** sugar cinnamon), to taste

Heat oven to 375°F. Wash potatoes thoroughly and pat dry with paper towels. Cut into 1-inch-thick wedges. Spray inside of a roasting pan or deep baking dish with cooking spray. Add cut potatoes and spray potatoes, too. Use hands to toss, making sure potatoes are well coated. Bake uncovered for about 20 minutes. Remove from oven and sprinkle with cinnamon. Return to oven for another 5–10 minutes. Shake pan once or twice during baking time. Remove and let cool, sprinkle with more cinnamon if desired.

Nutritional Information (per serving)
Calories: 115
Protein: 2.05 grams
Fat: trace
Carbohydrates: 22.25 grams (net carbohydrates; fiber deducted from total)
Fiber: 3.9 grams

GRAINS

BROWN RICE A LA PHANTOM

Whole grains are great low-glycemic carbohydrates that you should definitely incorporate into your eating plan. In this recipe I've paired organic long-grain brown rice with the best of all leafy greens—spinach—and that indispensable bulb, garlic, for a quick, delicious, and nutritious meal.

YIELD: APPROXIMATELY NINE 1-CUP SERVINGS

10-ounce package of fresh whole-leaf spinach

6 large cloves of garlic

2 cups (uncooked) organic long-grain brown rice

$1/4$ cup olive oil

Dash of salt, optional

Fresh ground black pepper, to taste

$1/2$ cup freshly grated Parmesan cheese

Rinse the spinach and let dry (dry completely before adding to hot oil). Roughly chop the garlic and set aside. Cook rice according to package directions (I recommend a rice cooker). Meanwhile, in a large, covered sauté pan, begin heating the olive oil. When oil is hot, add the garlic and sauté for a few minutes, constantly stirring so it doesn't burn. Reduce heat. Add the spinach, stirring to coat with the oil and cover. Let simmer for a few minutes, just enough to wilt the spinach. Add a dash of salt, if desired, and pepper to taste. Toss the spinach into the rice, sprinkle with Parmesan, and enjoy.

Nutritional Information (per serving)

Calories: 239

Protein: 6.42 grams

Fat: 8.90 grams

Carbohydrates: 31.60 grams (net carbohydrates;
                    fiber deducted from total)

Fiber: 2.16 grams

DESSERTS

BIG-BICEPS BERRY BLITZ

*Why settle for just plain fruit? You can easily mix several
compatible berries and fruits together, sprinkle with a little
lemon juice, and you've got a delicious, refreshing pick-me-up.*

YIELD: FOUR SERVINGS

$\frac{1}{2}$ cup blueberries

$\frac{1}{2}$ cup sliced strawberries

1 apple (red delicious preferred)

2 tablespoons fresh lemon juice

Stevia sweetener, optional

Wash and dry all fruit. Combine all ingredients in a covered container
and refrigerate about 2 hours before serving, but not much longer,
as the fruit can become mushy if left too long in the fridge.

Nutritional Information (per serving)

Calories: 35
Protein: 0.35 grams
Fat: 0.18 grams
Carbohydrates: 7.30 grams (net carbohydrates;
                fiber deducted from total)
Fiber: 1.70 grams

Darwin's Evolutionary Dessert

*This is a very simple, no-bake recipe that takes just minutes to prepare
and is sure to satisfy your sweet tooth.*

Yield: Approximately three dozen squares

6 ounces sugar-free chocolate chips,
or four 1$\frac{1}{2}$-ounce sugar-free dark-chocolate bars

$\frac{1}{2}$ cup natural peanut butter
(salted is recommended)

4 cups crisp soy cereal

Melt the chocolate over very low heat, or in a double boiler, stirring
constantly. Add the peanut butter and blend together well. Stir into the
cereal until it is well assimilated. Spray a 9 x 11-inch pan with nonstick
cooking spray, or line with aluminum foil. Press the mixture into the pan
and chill for several hours (3–4 hours is ideal). Cut into squares and store
covered in refrigerator until ready to serve.

Nutritional Information (per square)
  Calories: 55
  Protein: 1.70 grams
  Fat: 4.30 grams
  Carbohydrates: 2.65 grams (net carbohydrates;
                        fiber deducted from total)
  Fiber: 1.20 grams

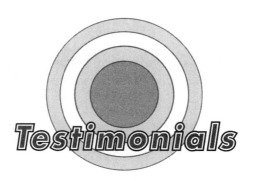

Testimonials

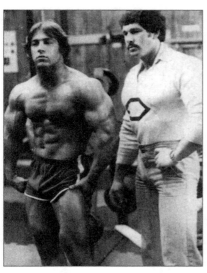

THERE ARE A FEW PEOPLE I RESPECT and Steve Michalik sits at the top of the list. He earned the respect I have for him—he trained and lived bodybuilding and he showed me what discipline and focus could do. This is something very few people will ever learn or understand, but I was blessed to have Steve Michalik in my life showing me the way. Steve always traveled a different path from others, and I learned to make my own path by following his example. He made me and my path truly unique, and although most people choose not to travel my path because it is bumpy and rough and not the easy way, the people who follow me have done well. The best path is not always the easiest to follow, but the easy way that others follow is not the best. Whether I am liked or disliked no longer matters. I have learned a lesson that Steve tried to teach me twenty years ago—there are so few friends, only acquaintances. Both Steve and I (thanks to Steve) have made our mark. There are many people who will remember us for years to come: the eccentric Michalik and his buddy DeFendis—two maniacs who did things their way. Both were champions who created champions. Both helped many people attain goals, and most of all . . . both did it with *passion*. Yes, Mr. America, we did good, regardless of what our critics think—critics are, after all, just wannabes who never had a plan themselves.

Be proud of who you are and what you have done for many people,

Michalik. You are, and will always be, great in my eyes! You have instilled in me the true meaning of *champion*! There are very few left. God bless you.

Love and respect, *John DeFendis*
Mr. USA, Trainer of the Year (nine times), author, celebrity personal trainer, developer of the ULTRA FIT Weight Loss Program, personal training director for more than 100 personal trainers, trainer at the Congressional Gym, Washington, D.C. As seen on *Hard Copy, 20/20, Good Morning America, NBC Sports, CNN, CBS News, The Joan Rivers Show*

I WISH I HAD MET STEVE MICHALIK BACK IN AUSTRALIA twenty years ago when I was a professional rugby player and track athlete. But I must warn you though—the information in this book is not for the faint hearted but for those who want results and the real truth in the maze of confusion called the fitness world.

You will need to open up your mind so that the prerecorded information stored there of the past trappings of falsehoods, misinformation, and confusion can be swept away by the exact training methods Steve has developed and tested for over forty-five years. But when you do start this adventure, your demons will doubt the truth as it collides with old information stored in your brain. So be aware, and get ready to confront the in-your-face laws of exercise and nutrition.

Steve Michalik is a surgeon in body symmetry and body mechanics, period. He stands alone. With nearly 50,000 hours of training and instruction, personal world titles, and making of champion physiques, he is without comparison. Don't bother rating others against him; I tried that and I fell flat on my butt with embarrassment, as did the rest of those who dared to challenge him.

In order to understand this declaration and his methodology, you will need to understand that Steve has one rule in his unwavering passion for the pursuit of truth in total fitness—no compromises.

The problem today is that the fitness and health industry is intent on confusing its customers and is no different from any other industry that sells its products through lies, half truths, partial information, and sugar-coated data. Magazines, athletes, and famous people endorse their products for a fee in an attempt to get you to believe their stories and buy their products. Add to that television ads and infomercials that spread that same "gerbil-on-a-spinning-wheel syndrome" of further lies—and now you have a real mess and a serious state of confusion concerning fitness and health. This opens the door for all types and brands of solutions that get you nowhere.

This is where Steve stands alone. He presents the whole "fitness and health" truth and nothing but the truth. He has cut out a six-lane freeway through the solid mountain of lies in the health and fitness arena.

What makes Steve different is that he came from an upbringing that could never have placed him in the bodybuilding and fitness field if he did not have drive, purpose, and a thirst for knowledge to get answers and achieve results. He spent years and years learning before the fitness industry went south. He was small, skinny, and didn't have the genetics to be a great champion. So he achieved his goals the hard way—by studying, taking notes, and experimenting with exercise techniques to get better results.

Let's face it, without the real basics of health and fitness, your nightmare of "not enough gains for the amount of work" will continue. Why? Well just take a look at our nation right now. We have the distinction of being the fattest country in the world. This is totally embarrassing! The most powerful nation on Earth doesn't have the ability to get the right information on fitness and health to the masses! We are all aware of the current trend to look great without sacrifice. Everyone wants a shortcut to a great physique and success. That ideology is the high road to disaster.

Back in the early days, fitness was simple and had some basic truths. The guys back in Steve's era didn't have high-tech machines or nutritional products. With the volumes of data and products available today, you really don't know if they work. Since you have no reference point to go by, you assume they do. However, Steve provides you with a reference point as well as the tools you need to put you in control of your destiny.

Steve Michalik comes from the school of raw, unadulterated "do or die" experience of testing for results; he discards anything that doesn't produce maximum gains. Then, he passes this tried-and-true data on to you, so it can become true for you as well; no other so-called true information can taint it or alter it in any way.

Coming from Down Under and having been trained by some of the most strict Rugby trainers and conditioning coaches for many years, I believed I had a fairly good background in fitness and health. I thought I knew about nutrition as it relates to performance. I was a track athlete in the 100M and 200M, and I never smoked or took any drugs. The knowledge I'd gained through my everyday experiences and the information I received from those who taught me was inaccurate and false in a way—I'd been led to believe I did not need to know any more. But deep down I knew that I did not know it all, and in a strange way, I knew that those around me did not know either. I needed to improve in this arena, but there was no person or body of knowledge with a proven track record at my disposal that I could turn too. I was in a hopeless situation with no way out.

When I met Steve, my life changed. I trusted him from day one and knew he would not lead me down the road I had been on before. He stripped me down to basics, and I got my butt kicked. But this was the price I was willing to pay to achieve the truth and results no matter the cost. The results I finally got were nothing short of miraculous. But more important, I had gained knowledge that makes me unshakable in this field and will keep me from ever becoming sidetracked again.

In truth, during this time, I felt ignorant for knowing little to nothing about body basics. I felt a little better when Olympic athletes from around the world sought out the "Steve experience." I was shocked to discover that even those who had access to unlimited knowledge of body mechanics and who had nutritional experts and strength coaches on their sides couldn't last five minutes doing the routines Steve had me doing. This feeling of triumph was short-lived, however. "Hell" was waiting for me as I progressed along my learning curve.

I spent the next four years doing to others what Steve taught me to do. I saw these people get result right before my eyes. This was the ultimate confirmation for me: witnessing the successes of others. Helping them achieve their goals brought me the joy of accomplishment.

There is only one way to get a job done and that is to do it right from the beginning by starting on the right road. This road will get you to the right place on time—it is wide open so you can see ahead of you, and there are no surprises. Although there may be other roads that seem to lead you down the right track, sooner or later, you will reach a dead end. You may never get back on track if your mind is filled with the disappointments that can block your desire to fulfill your dreams. When that happens, the demons in your head take over and you are "done for."

The road out of this mess has been built—all you need to do is follow it. When you can conquer the demons in your body, you can conquer the demons in your head. The battle awaits you, but now you can be assured of victory with knowledge on your side and with Steve, "the master," in your head, breaking down the barriers of your body. Take control, and you will never be the same again. You have been warned!

Joe Reaiche
Former Professional Rugby Player
Olympic Trainer and Health Expert

STEVE MICHALIK HAS BEEN MY PERSONAL TRAINER for the past fifteen years and I plan on keeping him for the next thirty. In fact, I am sure that the reason I'll be around and active for the next thirty years is because of the work I've done and will continue to do with Steve.

By the way, I'm sixty-six years old and would never trade how I look and feel today for how I looked and felt at the age of fifty-one when I first met Steve. Under his expert guidance I have been able to keep my weight down and increase and maintain muscle tone with a diet and exercise program that is both manageable and fun.

As President of the New York Mets, I have seen a host of training and diet regimes from more organizations and personal trainers than I'd like to remember. There is one reason why I've stood by Steve all these years: He is the best at what he does. And as Yogi Berra once said, "Baseball is ninety percent mental, the other half is physical." Besides improving my physical appearance and stamina, Steve's program has left me feeling more mentally alert and sharp.

In addition to my partnership in the Mets, as a partner in real estate, private equity, media, and investment business, also all the brands and charitable organizations I am involved with, I play an important leadership role in an organization that is more near and dear to me than anything else—my family. As a grandfather of a rapidly expanding clan, there is a lot to be done: babies to play with, son and sons-in-law to play tennis with, daughters and daughter-in-law to plan family outings and vacations with, etc. And right now, none of them can keep up with me!

Steve's approach is all about exercise, about finding the best in each client and helping each client to demand the best from him- or herself. He has taught me what I like to call "habits of health"—and because he can't be with me all the time, it is these habits that have kept me on his program all of these years. This philosophy is tried and true; indeed, Aristotle beat him when he said, "Excellence is an art won by training and habituation. We do not act rightly because we have virtue or excellence, but we rather have this because we have acted rightly. We are what we repeatedly do. Excellence, then, is not an act but a habit."

It is therefore with great confidence I recommend Steve Michalik and his approach to fitness and health to anyone looking to improve their quality of life.

Saul Katz
President of the New York Mets

gt;gt;

AS A BUSY, MIDDLE-AGED PHYSICIAN who spends her demanding days sitting and looking through a microscope, it can be difficult to maintain a trim figure, and this was starting to show. When I began searching for a mentor and inspiring trainer who would help me achieve my fitness goals, I found the best.

As a trained pathologist, I dissected Steve Michalik's training method from a distance. I watched him train bodybuilders and homemakers. I saw a caring, methodical, passionate, and very professional individual, as well as a demanding and disciplined teacher. I observed him not only train, but also motivate others to be the best they can be.

I approached Steve and discussed with him my dreams and goals. He instantly knew what I should do, and helped me formulate a dietary and exercise program that put me back on track in a time-efficient manner.

Steve's broad understanding of the human body's physiology and anatomy allows him to specifically target problem areas with a professional and knowledgeable approach. His workout is intense, but definitely not insane. But don't get me wrong, the training requires a strong-willed determination to endure multiple high-volume, fast-tempo reps, and vigorous nonstop supersets. Every muscle is worked hard and consistently. The muscles are overloaded by condensing more training into less time. The routine is completed in under an hour. It is a superb combination of aerobic and strength-training exercises.

His technique helped me drop pounds and lose inches off my waist, while developing a toned and muscular body. I became not only physically strong, but also emotionally balanced. My endurance and stamina have grown exponentially. Honest, hard-training sessions were the key to my progress.

It is with a profound sense of confidence that I recommend Steve Michalik's program to anyone who is seriously interested in losing weight and achieving a healthy lifestyle.

Patricia G. Tiscornia, M.D.

AS TIME MARCHES ON FOR ME, I can count on both hands all the individuals who have truly made a difference in my life. One of them is Steve Michalik, a soft-spoken giant of a person. It is odd that our paths would cross in the first place. I weight trained in one way or another for many years and could never fully understand the need for trainers. I have since taken a 180-degree turn from that belief. Steve changed all that for me and, from what I can see, for anyone else who is willing to listen. For the hard-core group that trains to be champions, Steve and his training methods seem to be heaven-sent. The mere mention of his name seems to bring smiles to the faces of the people he trains.

At my first meeting with him to elucidate my goals for weight training, he told me to look around the gym. Many of these people are here to train, he told me, but hardly any of them will ever benefit the way they could. I knew he was right because most of them hardly ever did change, myself included. It seemed that most people there were willing to put in the time, but not the energy required to make the strides they seemed to seek. Steve's approach was simple—intensity. For me, intensity has a different meaning than for Steve who became Mr. America and Mr. Universe thirty-plus years ago. Like the Nobel Prize, that is a feat achieved by only one individual a year, and, once attained, it can never be taken away. Steve would do it all over again if he could. He hates the mere mention of the word "can't," and he has honed his discipline to such a point that he still has the mental discipline to win any contest. He has taken his laser beam that was turned inward and began turning it outward to benefit those fortunate enough to cross his path.

Steve is great to train with. I have a long way to go, but I believe I am enjoying the journey more than the ultimate destination. Steve is able to size people up very fast and does not approach his clients with a cookie-cutter mentality. He definitely has tailored my program to my abilities, and he increases the level of intensity as I progress. The workout is strenuous but not time-consuming, and with my busy life, this is a real benefit. I can tell you that I feel like a million bucks after the workout.

Steve's moral compass points in all the right directions. His great spirituality, combined with his affability and huge base of knowledge, makes training more than just exercise. My mind has grown along with some skeletal muscle. If anyone wants to feel endorphins do their magic, spend forty-five minutes with Steve Michalik. I am proud to call him my trainer, friend, and mentor. His great ability to turn dreams into reality is awe-inspiring, and to those around him, infectious.

Alan Cohen, M.D.
American Academy of Physical Medicine and Rehabilitation

IN 1980, WHEN I WALKED INTO MR. AMERICA'S GYM, located in Farmingdale, New York, I was a twenty-two-year-old aerospace engineer who did not even shave yet. Behind the counter was the most muscular man I had ever seen. This person was Steve Michalik. He had muscles where I thought muscles did not exist. His enormous arms, chest, and shoulders gave him the appearance of an action figure, but it quickly became clear to me that his strongest muscles were not beneath his neck. Once he spoke, I knew he was not just another muscle-head. He communicated in such an articulate manner, with so much thought and sincerity. I remember asking him if working out with weights produced tightness, and he said, "Absolutely not. People who walk around like that are just acting." He said there was a study of Olympic athletes revealing that weight lifters were second behind gymnasts in terms of greatest flexibility, and both were extremely muscular. Now that I am a chiropractor, I share this story with all my patients when this question is asked of me.

Oddly enough, our paths crossed again twenty-four years later. I started to practice chiropractic in a gym where Steve trained people and got to know him personally when I eventually began treating him. We shared insightful conversations during that time and I had the opportunity to learn much about who he is. Steve trains many people, from amateurs to pros, for bodybuilding competitions. I've seen him take these individuals through a complete metamorphosis, naturally, in a matter of months. He has transformed the bodies of ordinary people into enviable, award-winning physiques. Steve has a remarkable talent for generating enthusiasm, happiness, self-discipline, and enjoyment among all of the athletes he trains. I never once heard a complaint or negative comment about all of the hard work and dieting they endure in order to optimize their training. A wise professor once said, "First arouse in the other person an eager want. He who can do this has the whole world with him. He who cannot walks a lonely way." I'd like to let you all know that Steve has the world with him.

One last story I would like to share is the lesson of the Wall of Fire. Steve explained that many times in life we get 80 percent of the way to our goal and we hit obstacles that appear insurmountable. This is what Buddhists call the Wall of Fire, he said, adding that most people usually give up at this point, but if you have the fortitude and discipline, you can walk through this wall and life will be more gratifying than you ever imagined. In Steve's life, there were many walls of fire he had to walk through and he always persevered so he would come out on the other side. I take this story and message with me every day. Steve has not only turned bodybuilding into a science, but also into a unique art form. I admire his creativity and genius.

Donald J. Wallace, D.C.

WHEN I MET STEVE, THE ONLY THING I HEARD him say was, "You need to bring your mind in line with your body." What did this mean? I wasn't sure, but one of my most memorable life experiences was about to begin. He said it would take three to four months to get my inner body to a level that would permit me to operate efficiently. He was right.

When the going was tough, he would say to me, "You can do it." He not only expects it, but he truly knows that you *can* do it. You learn that you must respect the master, and he proves it to you all the time.

At first, however, he didn't tell me about the personal growth I would experience through sharing our respective life journeys. This personal expansion came not only through my muscle, but through gaining a new mental awareness as well. A man of worldliness had entered my life, and the opportunity to work with him is a life experience that will stay with me for a long time to come. I now know what he meant when he said, "You need to bring your mind in line with your body."

Lloyd J. Streisand
Vice President and Senior Loan Officer
The Streisand Team at Sterling National Mortgage

SINCE THE FALL OF 1990, AT LEAST ONCE A DAY, I have thanked Steve Michalik for somehow changing, or rather saving, my life. I first met Steve at a gym in Port Washington, New York. At the time, I was suffering from sarcoidosis, an autoimmune disease that was attacking my lungs and had reduced my lung function to 45 percent of normal capacity—the disease causes scar tissue to form around the lungs and makes it difficult to breathe (to say the least).

Before I met Steve, I had never exercised a day in my life. I was never much interested in sports and weight training (those words were not even in my vocabulary). The conventional medical treatment for sarcoid was prednisone, and I had been taking it for more than a year and not getting any better. I was physically sick, depressed, fat, tired from the medication, and not optimistic about the future because I wasn't getting any positive results from the drug therapy. To the contrary, I saw myself showing more and more damaging physical signs of prolonged prednisone use. For reasons I was not aware of at the time, I dragged myself to the gym, probably figuring I had nothing to lose anyway.

Everyone who knows Steve has heard stories about how tough he is in the gym. I have to say, though, that with me, he was the most inspiring force imaginable. Within six weeks of training with Steve, suffering through two painful exercise sessions a week with him, and following his dietary and nutritional guidance, my lung function tested in the 90 percent range—an almost normal lung function.

There were times in those weeks when I would actually pass out and Steve would catch me by the seat of my pants; times when I would turn green and make mad dashes to the bathroom to throw up. But Steve's nurturing and caring kept me coming back again and again for more and more training. I never once entertained the thought of quitting. I was seeing and feeling results. I saw that Steve was better for me than the North Shore doctors who were treating me.

After the lung-function test, the doctor who told me the results had two things to say. The first was that the change in my lung function must have been a "spontaneous remission" of the disease. The second was that maybe it was time to reduce the prednisone. I very proudly told him I had been working out with Steve for the previous six weeks and had stopped taking the medication the first day I met Steve.

I do not look like a bodybuilder. I don't have Popeye-looking bulges. But I'm healthy and I'm strong. My mental focus is better than it has ever been. I trained with Steve for about two years. My suit size initially went from a 42 regular down to a 39 from fat loss. Then I started growing. I blew past a size 42 and I remember the beautiful suit I treated myself to when I measured in at size 44, a suit that got small on me very quickly. All of a sudden I had a 46-inch chest and shoulders that didn't droop. Nobody would confuse me with the sickly man who could barely walk when I first presented myself at the gym.

I thank Steve for being there for me in my years of need, and for leading me out of the darkness of illness and into the beauty of physical well-being.

Larry Tallis
Little Neck, New York

I MET STEVE MICHALIK SEVERAL YEARS AGO when I was growing frustrated by the lack of results with the usual body-training methods. I am a busy professional with limited time for exercise and was looking for somebody who would help me reach my goals in the most efficient way.

The workout method developed by Steve has helped transform my body in unimaginable ways. It is a method that focuses on high reps and proper technique, done at a quick and constant tempo. This practice helps improve flexibility and strength while defining and toning the body.

Steve has an extensive knowledge of human physiology, something I can appreciate as a physician. He knows just by looking at you the appropriate weight you should be lifting. He helps control each of your movements, allowing you to train without sustaining injuries, and every workout is different. There is not the monotony usually experienced with other training routines. This is essential because you always look forward to the next session instead of dreading it.

On a personal level, Steve is pleasant, energetic, and compassionate. Despite his incredible personal achievements, he is a down-to-earth and caring individual.

Following his program and a healthy diet, I was able to lose inches off my waist and decrease my body fat while increasing muscle mass. These results gave me a more defined and muscular body than I ever had before.

I can say with the utmost confidence that Steve's program is one of the best methods anywhere for getting into shape and redefining the body and mind. I recommend it to everybody without reservations.

Daniel H. Wasserman, M.D.

WHEN I MET STEVE MICHALIK IN MARCH of 2004, I was just getting back into the gym after taking a year off—just another of the low swings in my yo-yo dieting/fitness mode that I had blindly been following for years.

I was horribly out of shape (again), weighing over 160 pounds. I had been close to 200 several years earlier, and was on my way back up there again. My eating habits were a mess and I had recently quit smoking (again), so I was gaining body fat much faster than usual. My self-esteem was nonexistent, and quite honestly, I felt like crap.

Well, everything happens for a reason. It was destiny that actually got me the courage to call Steve (I never hired a trainer before) and ask him for help. And it was the beginning of a beautiful friendship.

It's very hard to put into words how I feel about Steve. How do you express your gratitude for someone who has taken you from a monotonous, lackluster, apathetic, unhealthy, boring existence to a vibrant, exciting, energetic, happy, and healthy lifestyle? Not to mention being groomed to become a top-ranked natural bodybuilder—all in a *few short months*. On September 11, 2004, at age forty-one, I competed for the first time, weighing in at 123 pounds, with less than 9 percent body fat.

And that's just scratching the surface. Steve has taught me so much about life. The apparent physical benefits pale in comparison to the psychological strength and well-being that he instilled in me. I now understand what Steve meant when he said, "The way out is the way through," and I live it every day. You can, too.

> Thank you, Steve, for being you.
> For sharing your incredible knowledge.
> For teaching me to be strong,
> both physically and mentally.
> For helping me to break
> down the barriers and see clearly.
> For helping me to disagree and go free.
>
> And especially,
> for being my most treasured friend.

Emy Bradley

STEVE MICHALIK CHANGED MY LIFE FOREVER. As a freshman in high school, I was completely out of shape. I played three different sports, but even with all my activity, I couldn't lose any weight. I was close to 300 pounds and I wore size 46 jeans. I couldn't understand why, even with so much activity, I was still so heavy. So I decided to see a professional. That was when I met Steve.

Steve knew just what I needed to do and we began working together three times a week. Little by little, I began losing the weight. I couldn't believe it when, just four months later, I was down to 180 pounds and into size 32 jeans. Right then I felt I owed Steve the world. I couldn't have been happier. But we didn't stop there. In January 2004, Steve asked me to give him eight months so he could make me a champion bodybuilder. His words were more than I could grasp, but I believed in him, so of course I said yes.

The next eight months were like boot camp. Every time I thought I had Steve figured out, he would come at me from a new direction. My body began developing faster than I could have ever imagined. On September 11, 2004, I competed in my first all-natural bodybuilding competition. I thought I was dreaming when I was awarded the gold trophy in the teenage division. Not only was my body superior to my opponents, but with Steve's guidance, my posing, my routine, and my music made everyone else look unprepared.

Steve took me from a size 46, weighing 300 pounds, to a size 29, weighing 169 pounds, with 2.8 percent body fat. I owe everything to Steve and don't know where I'd be without him.

Anthony Thomasello

STEVE MICHALIK IS A VERY UNIQUE INDIVIDUAL, and a one-of-a-kind trainer who possesses characteristics other people don't. When Steve talks, everyone around him will stop what they're doing to hear him speak. He has the ability to motivate a person to believe there is nothing they can't accomplish. And Steve does not just teach training and nutrition, he teaches people about life, teaches them how to expect the best from themselves and persevere through tough times, and teaches that being average is not enough, you must want more.

I had been weight training for several years before I met Steve, but I now consider all that training beforehand a waste of time. His principles work because he makes you train with an intensity you never thought possible. Your mind says, I can't do any more, then you do twenty-five more reps. I have never felt so alive, and I owe it all to Steve. With his guidance, I have been able to reach goals I never thought possible. I not only lost a significant amount of fat and replaced it with pounds of muscle, but with his help I have become a bodybuilder and I am mentally and physically stronger than I ever thought possible. He is extremely knowledgeable because he has been through it all, and has conquered every barrier he ever came up against. Steve's influence has changed my life for the better. I now know that I have what it takes to conquer physical and mental barriers in the gym **and** in life. With the knowledge and motivation Steve has given me, I know I can accomplish anything I set my mind to.

Frank Thomasello

AFTER A LONG AND PROUD CAREER as a registered nurse, marriage, home, and family made it necessary for me to take an extended sabbatical from my beloved profession. As demanding as my nursing career was, I've found that my current responsibilities require a far greater amount of time than I could possibly have predicted. There seems to be time for everything and everyone but myself. Exercise, especially, was put on the back burner. I was another victim of the eternal excuse—until the day I looked in the mirror and saw someone I didn't know looking back at me. Suddenly something clicked. This wasn't what I wanted. My family deserved better. *I* deserved better. Within a few days of that life-altering moment, I joined a gym. I would work out three to four days a week—not bad, right? A few months passed, but that same person was still in the mirror. What was I doing wrong? I was exercising and I had changed my eating habits (somewhat), so what was the problem? I worked harder at the gym, increased my cardio, and hired a personal trainer. Another year passed. The results—nada, zilch, nothing—were highly frustrating.

Then I met Steve Michalik. I thought to myself, "Wow, he looks great. He probably knows what he's doing." Little did I know how much of an understatement that was. I approached him one day and asked if he could help me, and he said he would.

Steve isn't your run-of-the-mill bodybuilder/trainer. When you enter into Michalik madness, you enter a place where very few have gone before. In just a few short weeks, I began to see drastic changes in myself and my body. After all the previous months of frustration, I couldn't believe my results. Steve doesn't just run your body through a physical routine, he watches, listens, and learns, from both verbal and nonverbal communication. His methods are revolutionary. As a registered nurse, I felt I had a firm understanding of how the body works, but Steve gave me a real education. He teaches you about yourself as well as your body, and the combination is indeed life altering.

There are still only twenty-four hours in a day, but besides the fact that Steve's routines require a fraction of the time I was investing before, I now have the energy, strength, and knowledge to handle my daily tasks more efficiently. Most importantly, that awful person in the mirror has finally gone.

Linda Bove, R.N.

STEVE MICHALIK IS BY FAR THE BIGGEST POSITIVE influence in my life. Steve has made me a better person. He has inspired me to be the best at whatever I choose to do in my life. He has taught me values and shown me there is no limit to what I can accomplish. Nothing is impossible with confidence and positive thinking. You are what you think. He has taught me to believe in myself and to never let any negative forces affect my life.

His Intensity/Insanity workouts have improved my physical being *and* my spiritual, social, emotional, and mental health. Steve taught me how training is 90 percent mental. The body is not meant to have a great build, so it will turn to survival mode and fight you every step of the way. When I'm training and reach the point of failure, I know that the pain is all in my head, not my muscles. When I'm battling an injury or stress in my life, I refuse to let it bring me down. I stay focused and clear. Steve's philosophy has helped me understand what barriers are and how to "disagree and go free." Because of Steve, I've become a more powerful person, both in and out of the gym.

Steve brings new meaning to the word "intensity." Steve showed me what it means to train hard. He challenges your mind as well as your muscles. There is nothing I look forward to more than the challenge of one of his workouts. No one has ever pushed me to the level Steve has. Just his presence makes me train harder. Every workout is an opportunity to learn more about myself and an opportunity to improve mentally and physically. Steve taught me that it is not how *long* you train, but how hard and intensely. Failure is not an option.

Working with Steve has been an incredible experience. Each day I look forward to training hard and increasing my knowledge. Steve has steered me in the right direction so I can lead a powerful and productive lifestyle, helping others along the way. Learning from the best, I look forward to making him proud by encouraging others to reach their goals so they can truly live the life. To have the opportunity to be trained and guided by Steve Michalik is an honor. I am thankful every day to have someone like him in my life.

T. J. Lynch
Bodybuilder, trainer

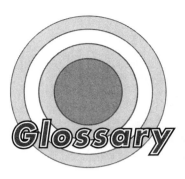

Glossary

Aerobic. Any activity that requires the utilization of oxygen in order to strengthen the cardiopulmonary system.

Allowance. The amount of a nutrient needed by a healthy person of a certain age, sex, and weight. Extra stress or ailments may cause nutritional needs to be increased above normal allowances.

Anabolism. The constructive part of metabolism involving building up of molecules and tissues.

Anaerobic. Without the presence of oxygen. Exercises designed for purposes other than strengthening the cardiopulmonary system.

Balance. Maintaining proper levels of all nutrients in the diet, including proper levels of carbohydrates, fats, and proteins.

Calorie. A unit of energy from food. 1 gram carbohydrate = 4 calories; 1 gram protein = 4 calories; 1 gram fat = 9 calories.

Catabolism. The destructive part of metabolism involving breaking down complex molecules into simple molecules.

Chemical bonds. Basic structures in chemistry that make up the different elements throughout the universe, including those in the body, such as H_2O.

Cleans. Exercises performed by lifting dumbbells or barbells from the floor to your shoulders.

Enzymes. Any of the numerous proteins produced by the body that function as biochemical catalysts.

Essential nutrient. A substance needed by the body, which cannot be manufactured within the body or made by intestinal bacteria. For example, vitamin C is an essential nutrient for humans, but not for animals.

Gram. A weight equal to about one twenty-eighth of an ounce. For example, a nickel coin weighs 5 grams.

Homeostasis. A state of equilibrium (balance) between the interrelated functions and elements of the body.

Irritability. The inflammation of a muscle due to a response to stimuli (weight training).

Microgram (mcg). One millionth of a gram. Micrograms are used to measure biotin, vitamin B_{12}, and trace minerals, such as copper and iodine.

Milligram (mg). One thousandth of a gram. Milligrams are used to measure water-soluble vitamins, as well as minerals, such as calcium, iron, magnesium, phosphorus, potassium, and sodium.

Minerals. Minerals are elements that originate in the earth. Most minerals in the diet come indirectly from animal sources or directly from plants. They are also present in the water, but this varies with geographic location. Because the mineral content of the soil varies geographically, minerals from plant sources may also vary from place to place.

Nutrient. A chemical substance in food that provides energy, forms new body components, or assists in the functioning of various body processes.

Nutrition. The study of the nutrients needed by living beings. Good nutrition means obtaining and balancing all the nutrients in your daily diet, often using supplements to supply those nutrients not available in foods.

Oxygen debt. This is the precursor to muscular failure. If breathing becomes difficult while doing fat-burning exercises, you are experiencing oxygen debt. In this condition, a body is working muscles and burning sugar, *not* fat.

Phytochemicals. These are chemicals produced by plants. Generally, the term is used to describe chemicals that are not essential nutrients, but may affect health.

Phytonutrients. Plant nutrients that are derived directly from the plants themselves, rather than synthetic duplications.

Stress. Anything that places strain on the nervous and glandular systems of the body. Stress may be internal (from ailments to malnutrition) or external (from environmental factors).

Supplements. Nutrients taken in addition to your regular food. Supplements may be in the form of liquids, pills, or powders. Some foods are considered supplemental; they are not in the ordinary diet but can be used to add nutrients to your diet.

Units. A measurement for the activity or strength of fat-soluble vitamins. There are international units (IU) and United States Pharmacopoeia units (USP units). (Both are, for practical purposes, the same.)

Vitamin. An organic compound obtained through diet or supplements that regulates metabolic functions of the body.

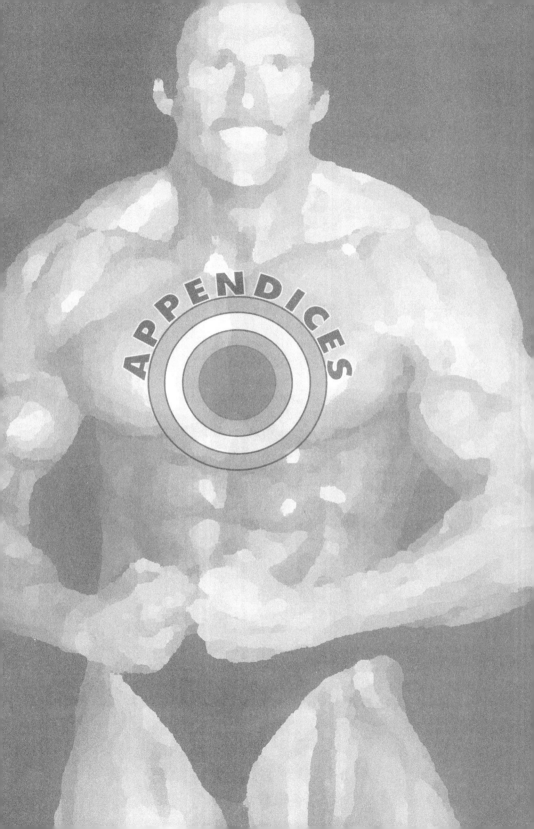

APPENDICES

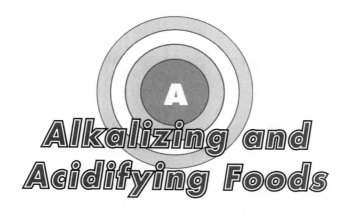

Alkalizing and Acidifying Foods

ALKALIZING FOODS

Fruits

Apple
Apricot
Avocado
Banana (high glycemic)
Berries
Cantaloupe
Cherries
Currant
Dates
Figs
Grape
Grapefruit
Lemon
Lime
Melon, honeydew
Nectarine
Orange
Peach
Pear
Pineapple
Tangerine
Tomato
Tropical fruit
Watermelon

Proteins

Almond
Chestnut
Chicken breast
Cottage cheese
Eggs
Flaxseed
Millet
Nuts
Pumpkin seeds
Sprouted seeds
Squash seeds
Sunflower seeds
Tempeh (fermented)
Tofu (fermented)
Yogurt
Whey protein powder

Seasonings and Spices

Chili pepper
Cinnamon
Curry
Ginger

Herbs
Miso
Mustard
Sea salt
Tamari

Sweeteners

Stevia

Vegetables

Alfalfa
Asparagus
Barley grass
Beets
Broccoli
Brussels sprouts
Cabbage
Carrot
Cauliflower
Celery
Chard
Chlorella
Collard greens
Cucumber
Dandelions

Edible flowers
Eggplant
Fermented vegetables
Garlic
Kale
Kohlrabi
Lettuce
Mushrooms
Mustard greens
Nightshade vegetables
Onions
Parsnips (high glycemic)
Peas
Peppers
Pumpkin
Rutabaga
Spirulina
Sprouts
Squash
Watercress
Wheat grass
Wild greens

ALKALIZING FOODS (continued)

Vegetables, Asian

Daikon
Dandelion root
Dulse
Kombu
Maitake mushrooms
Nori
Reishi mushrooms

Sea vegetables
Shiitake mushrooms
Umeboshi
Wakame

Other

Alkaline antioxidant
  water

Apple cider vinegar
Bancha tea
Bee pollen
Dandelion tea
Fresh fruit juice
Ginseng tea
Green juices
Green tea

Herbal tea
Kombucha
Lecithin granules
Mineral water
Organic milk
  (unpasteurized)
Probiotic cultures
Vegetable juices

ACIDIFYING FOODS

Alcohol

Beer
Hard liquor
Spirits
Wine

Beans and Legumes

Almond milk
Black beans
Chickpeas
Green peas
Kidney beans
Lentils
Lima beans
Pinto beans
Red beans
Rice milk
Soy milk
Soybeans
White beans

Dairy

Butter
Cheese, cow
Cheese, goat

Cheese, processed
Cheese, sheep
Milk

Drugs and Chemicals

Drugs, medicinal
Drugs, psychedelic
Herbicides
Pesticides

Fats and Oils

Avocado oil
Canola oil
Corn oil
Flax oil
Hemp seed oil
Lard
Olive oil
Safflower oil
Sesame oil
Sunflower oil

Fruits

Cranberries

Grains

Amaranth
Barley
Buckwheat
Corn
Hemp seed flour
Kamut
Oats (rolled)
Quinoa
Rice (all)
Rice cakes
Rye
Spelt
Wheat
Wheat cakes

Nuts and Butters

Brazil nuts
Cashews
Peanuts
Peanut butter
Pecans
Tahini
Walnuts

Pasta, White

Macaroni
Noodles
Spaghetti

Proteins, Animal

Beef
Carp
Clams
Fish
Lamb
Lobster
Mussels
Oyster
Pork
Rabbit
Salmon
Scallops
Shrimp
Tuna
Turkey
Venison

Other

Distilled vinegar
Potatoes
Wheat germ

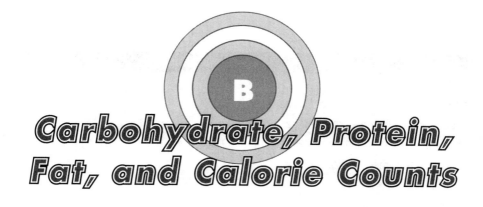

Carbohydrate, Protein, Fat, and Calorie Counts

All nutritional information in this appendix is retrieved from the USDA National Nutrient Database for Standard Reference.

Food Item	Carbs (g)	Protein (g)	Fat (g)	Calories
Beverages, Nonalcoholic				
Carbonated Drinks (12 fl oz)				
Club soda	0	0	0	0
Cola	3	0	0	13
Cream soda	4	0	0	16
Ginger ale	3	0	0	10
Grape soda	3	0	0	13
Lemon-lime	3	0	0	12
Orange	4	0	0	15
Root beer	3	0	0	13
Tonic water	3	0	0	10
Chocolate Drinks				
Chocolate drink, commercial, 1 percent fat (1 cup, 250 g)	25	8	3	158
Chocolate drink, commercial, 2 percent fat (1 cup, 250 g)	24	8	8	176
Chocolate drink, commercial, whole milk (1 cup, 250 g)	24	8	8	208
Cocoa mix, Nestlé, Carnation with marshmallows (1 envelope)	24	1	1	112
Cocoa mix, Nestlé, Carnation, no sugar added (1 envelope)	8	4	0	55

Food Item	Carbs (g)	Protein (g)	Fat (g)	Calories
Coffee				
Coffee, brewed with tap water (1 fl oz)	0	0	0	1
Cappuccino with whole milk (12 fl oz)	11	7	7	140
Latte with low-fat milk (12 fl oz)	17	12	6	170
Latte with skim milk (12 fl oz)	17	12	6	120
Juices, Fruit				
Apple, canned or bottled, unsweetened (4 fl oz)	14.5	0.1	0.1	58
Apple, unsweetened (1 fl oz)	4	0	0	15
Cranberry juice cocktail (4 fl oz)	18.2	0	0.1	72
Grape juice, canned or bottled, unsweetened (1 fl oz)	5	0	0	20
Grape juice, unsweetened (1 fl oz)	5	0	0	20
Grapefruit juice, canned, unsweetened (1 fl oz)	3	0	0	12
Grapefruit juice, white, raw (1 fl oz)	3	0	0	12
Lemon juice, raw (1 fl oz)	3	0	0	8
Lime juice, raw (1 fl oz)	3	0	0	8
Orange juice, canned, unsweetened (1 fl oz)	3	0	0	13
Orange juice, raw (1 fl oz)	3	0	0	14
Pineapple juice, canned, unsweetened (1 fl oz)	4	0	0	17
Prune juice (1 fl oz)	5	0	0	23
Milk				
Skim (8 fl oz)	12	7	0	86
1 percent (8 fl oz)	12	7	2	105
2 percent (8 fl oz)	12	7	5	125
Tea				
Brewed with tap water (1 fl oz)	0	0	0	0
Herbal (except chamomile) (1 fl oz)	0	0	0	0
Iced, diet, Nestea (8 fl oz)	1.2	0	0	3
Iced, sweetened, Nestea (8 fl oz)	18	0	0	65
Iced, lemon, Snapple sweetened (8 fl oz)	22.6	0	0	88
Iced, lemon, Snapple diet (8 fl oz)	8.4	0	0	21
Water (8 fl oz)	0	0	0	0

Food Item	Carbs (g)	Protein (g)	Fat (g)	Calories
Beverages, Alcoholic				
Beer (12 fl oz)	13.2	1.1	0	146
Beer, light (12 fl oz)	4.6	0.7	0	99
Hard liquor: bourbon, gin, rum, vodka, and so on, any proof (1 fl oz)	0	0	0	82
Wine, red (3$\frac{1}{2}$ fl oz)	1.8	0.2	0	74
Wine, white (3$\frac{1}{2}$ fl oz)	0.8	0.1	0	70
Wine cooler (3$\frac{1}{2}$ fl oz)	5.9	0.1	0	49
Breads				
Bagels				
Cinnamon-raisin (1 oz, 28 g)	15	3	1	77
Oat bran (1 oz, 28 g)	15	3	0	77
Plain (1 oz, 28 g)	15	3	1	77
Plain with onion, poppy, sesame (1 oz, 28 g)	15	3	1	77
Biscuits				
Mixed grain, baked (1 oz)	15	2	2	85
Plain or buttermilk (1 oz)	13	2	4	102
Bread Sticks				
Plain (1 small stick, approximately 4$\frac{1}{2}$ inches long)	3	1	1	21
English Muffin				
Plain (1)	26.2	4.3	1.5	139
Sourdough (1)	25.8	4.3	1	132
Whole wheat (1)	26.7	5.8	1.4	134
Muffins (2 oz)				
Banana nut (1)	29	3	7	190
Blueberry (1)	27.2	3.1	3.7	157
Bran (1)	23.7	4	7.3	163
Corn (1)	28.9	3.4	4.8	173
Oat Bran (1)	11	3	1	66
Pita				
White (1 oz, 4-inch diameter)	16	3	0	77
Whole wheat (1 oz, 4-inch diameter)	15	3	1	74

Food Item	Carbs (g)	Protein (g)	Fat (g)	Calories
Rolls				
Croissant (1)	20	4	8	170
Dinner (1)	14.3	2.4	2.1	85
Hamburger (1)	21.7	3.6	3.1	129
White, hard (1)	14.9	2.8	1.2	83
Whole wheat (1)	14.5	2.5	1.3	75
Breads, Assorted				
Banana, prepared with margarine from recipe (1 oz, 28 g)	15	1	3	91
Cornbread (1 oz, 28 g)	20	2	3	117
Egg (1 oz, 28 g)	13	3	2	80
French, sourdough, or Vienna (1 oz, 28 g)	15	3	1	77
Irish soda bread (1 oz, 28g)	16	2	1	81
Pumpernickel (1 slice)	12	2	1	65
Pumpkin (1 oz, 28 g)	14	1	4	93
Rye, reduced calorie (1 slice)	9	2	1	47
Stuffing, dry mix, prepared (1 oz)	6	1	3	50
Wheat, reduced calorie (1 slice)	10	2	0	46
White, reduced calorie (1 slice)	10	2	0	48
Dairy and Eggs				
Butter				
With salt (1 tablespoon)	0	0	11	100
Without salt (1 tablespoon)	0	0	11	100
Cheese				
American, pasteurized (1 oz)	2	6	7	92
Blue (1 cubic inch)	0	4	5	60
Camembert (1 oz, 28 g)	0	6	7	84
Cheddar (1 cup, 132 g)	1	33	44	532
Cottage, 1 percent fat (4 oz, 113 g)	3	14	1	81
Cottage, 2 percent fat (4 oz, 113 g)	5	16	2	102
Cream cheese, fat-free (100 g)	6	14	1	96
Cream cheese (1 tbs, 14 g)	0	1	5	49
Feta (1 oz, 28 g)	1	4	6	74

Food Item	Carbs (g)	Protein (g)	Fat (g)	Calories
Goat, hard (1 oz, 28 g)	1	9	10	127
Goat, semi-soft (1 oz, 28 g)	1	6	8	102
Goat, soft (1 oz, 28 g)	0	5	6	75
Gouda (1 oz, 28 g)	1	7	8	100
Gruyère, shredded (1 cup, 108 g)	0	32	35	446
Limburger (1 oz, 28 g)	0	6	8	92
Monterey Jack, shredded (1 cup, 113 g)	1	27	34	421
Mozzarella, part skim (1 cup, 113 g)	1	7	4	71
Mozzarella, whole milk (1 cubic inch, 18 g)	1	5	6	79
Muenster, shredded (1 cup, 113 g)	1	26	34	416
Neufchatel (1 oz, 28 g)	1	3	6	73
Parmesan, grated (1 tbs, 5 g)	0	2	2	23
Parmesan, hard (1 cubic inch, 10 g)	0	4	3	39
Parmesan, shredded (1 tbs, 5 g)	0	2	1	21
Pimento, pasteurized process, diced (1 cup, 140 g)	3	31	43	525
Provolone (1 oz, 28 g)	1	7	8	98
Ricotta, part skim (1 oz, 28 g)	1	3	2	39
Ricotta, whole milk (1/2 cup, 124 g)	4	14	16	216
Romano (1 oz, 28 g)	1	9	8	108
Roquefort (1 oz, 28 g)	1	6	9	103
Swiss, diced (1 cup, 132 g)	4	37	36	496
Eggs				
Egg white, raw, fresh (1 large egg, 33 g)	0	4	0	17
Substitute, liquid (1 tablespoon, 16 g)	0	2	0	13
Substitute, powder (0.35 oz, 10 g)	2	6	1	44
Whole egg, hard boiled (1 tablespoon, 8 g)	0	1	1	12
Whole egg, raw (1 extra large, 58 g)	1	7	6	86
Milk Products				
Buttermilk, fluid, cultured from skim milk (1 oz, 31 g)	2	1	0	12
Cream, fluid, half and half (1 tablespoon, 15 g)	1	0	2	20
Cream, fluid, heavy whipping (1 cup, 120 g)	4	2	44	414

Food Item	Carbs (g)	Protein (g)	Fat (g)	Calories
Cream, fluid, light whipping (1 cup, 120 g)	4	2	37	350
Eggnog (1 fl oz, 32 g)	4	1	2	43
Milk shake, chocolate (8 fl oz, 224 g)	48	8	8	264
Milk shake, vanilla (8 fl oz, 224 g)	40	8	8	248
Sour cream, cultured (1 oz, 28 g)	2	1	6	58
Whipped topping, pressurized (1 tbs, 3 g)	0	0	1	8
Fruits				
Apples, raw with skin (1 cup, 110 g)	17	0	0	65
Apples, raw without skin (1 cup, 110 g)	17	0	0	63
Applesauce, sweetened (1 cup, 255 g)	51	0	0	194
Applesauce, unsweetened (1 cup, 255 g)	27	0	0	105
Apricots, raw (1 cup, 155 g)	17	2	0	74
Avocados, raw (1 cup, 150 g)	11	3	23	242
Bananas, raw (1 cup, 150 g)	35	2	0	138
Blackberries, raw (1 cup, 144 g)	19	1	0	75
Blueberries, raw (1 cup, 145 g)	20	1	0	81
Cherries, sweet, raw (1 cup, 117 g)	20	1	1	84
Cranberries, raw (1 cup, 95 g)	12	0	0	47
Cranberry sauce, canned, sweetened (1-1/2-inch-thick slice)	22	0	0	86
Dates, natural and dry (1 date, 8 g)	6	0	0	22
Figs, raw (1 medium, 2½ inches diameter, 50 g)	10	1	0	37
Fruit cocktail, canned, light syrup (1 cup, 242 g)	36	0	0	138
Grapes, raw, American type (1 grape, 2 g)	0	0	0	1
Grapefruit, pink, red, and white (approximately 4½ inches diameter, 166 g)	13	2	0	53
Guavas, common, raw (1 fruit, 90 g)	11	1	1	46
Kiwi, raw, without skin (1 large fruit, 91 g)	14	1	0	56
Lemons, raw, without peel (1 fruit, 2½ inches diameter, 58 g)	5	1	0	17
Limes, raw (1 fruit, 2 inches diameter, 67 g)	7	1	0	20
Mangos, raw (1 cup, 165 g)	28	2	0	107
Melons, cantaloupe, raw (1 cup, 160 g)	13	2	0	56

Food Item	Carbs (g)	Protein (g)	Fat (g)	Calories
Melons, honeydew, raw (1 cup, 160 g)	15	0	0	60
Nectarines, raw (1 fruit, 136 g)	16	2	0	67
Olives, ripe, canned, small to large (4 g)	0	0	0	5
Oranges, raw, all commercial varieties (1 cup, 180 g)	22	2	0	85
Papayas, raw (1 cup, 140 g)	14	1	0	55
Peaches, raw (2 3/4 inches diameter)	17	2	0	68
Pears, raw (1 cup, 165 g)	25	0	0	97
Pineapple, raw (1 cup, 155 g)	19	0	0	76
Plums, raw (1 fruit, 66 g)	9	1	1	36
Prunes, dried, stewed, without added sugar (1 cup, 248 g)	69	2	0	265
Raisins, seeded (1 cup, 145 g)	113	4	1	429
Raspberries, raw (1 cup, 123 g)	15	1	1	60
Strawberries, raw (1 cup, 152 g)	11	2	0	46
Tangerines, mandarin oranges, raw (2 1/2 inches diameter, 98 g)	11	1	0	43
Watermelon, raw (1 cup, 152 g)	11	2	0	49
Fish and Shellfish				
Fish				
Anchovy (1 anchovy, 4 g)	0	1	0	8
Bass, striped (3 oz, 85 g)	0	20	3	105
Bluefish (3 oz, 85 g)	0	22	4	135
Caviar, black and red (1 tablespoon, 16 g)	1	4	3	40
Gefilte fish, commercial (1 piece, 42 g)	3	4	1	35
Halibut, Atlantic and Pacific (3 oz, 85 g)	0	23	3	119
Herring, Atlantic, boneless (1 oz, 28 g)	3	4	5	73
Mackerel, Atlantic (3 oz, 85 g)	0	20	15	223
Monkfish (3 oz, 85 g)	0	16	2	82
Salmon, wild (3 oz, 85 g)	0	19	9	175
Sardine, Atlantic, canned in oil (1 oz, 28 g)	0	7	3	58
Swordfish (3 oz, 85 g)	0	21	4	132
Trout, rainbow, farmed (1 fillet, 71 g)	0	17	5	120
Tuna, light, canned in oil (3 oz, 85 g)	0	8	2	55
Tuna, light, canned in water (3 oz, 28 g)	0	7	0	32

Food Item	Carbs (g)	Protein (g)	Fat (g)	Calories
Shellfish				
Alaskan king crab (3 oz, 85 g)	0	16	2	82
Blue crab (1 cup, 118 g)	0	24	2	120
Clams, breaded and fried (3 oz, 85 g)	9	12	9	172
Clams (3 oz, 85 g)	4	22	2	126
Lobster (3 oz, 85 g)	1	17	1	83
Oyster, farmed (6 medium, 59 g)	4	4	1	47
Scallops, breaded and fried (2 large, 31 g)	3	6	3	67
Scallops (3 oz, 85 g)	9	11	0	84
Shrimp, breaded and fried (4 large, 30 g)	3	6	4	7
Shrimp (1 oz, 28 g)	0	6	1	34
Squid, fried (3 oz, 85g)	7	15	6	149
Meat				
Beef				
Brisket, all grades, braised (3 oz, 85 g)	0	21	24	309
Beef ribs, braised (3 oz, 85 g)	0	19	36	400
Chuck, blade roast, all grades, braised (3 oz, 85 g)	0	23	22	293
Porterhouse steak, all grades, broiled (3 oz, 85 g)	0	20	21	273
T-bone steak, all grades, broiled (3 oz, 85 g)	0	23	9	173
Tenderloin, all grades, broiled (3 oz, 85 g)	0	21	17	247
Top loin, all grades, broiled (3 oz, 85 g)	0	25	8	176
Top sirloin, all grades, broiled (3 oz, 85 g)	0	24	13	219
Lamb and Veal				
Lamb, domestic, composite of cuts trimmed to $1/4$-inch fat, choice (3 oz, 85 g)	0	10	50	498
Lamb, cubed for stew or kabob, leg or shoulder, trimmed to $1/4$-inch fat (3 oz, 85 g)	0	24	6	158
Lamb, leg, shank and sirloin, trimmed to $1/4$-inch fat (3 oz, 85 g)	0	24	7	162
Veal, breast (1 oz, 28 g)	0	3	15	146
Veal, ground, broiled (3 oz, 85 g)	0	20	7	146
Veal, cubed for stew, leg or shoulder (3 oz, 85 g)	0	30	3	160

Food Item	Carbs (g)	Protein (g)	Fat (g)	Calories
Pork				
Bacon (3 medium slices)	0	6	9	109
Canadian bacon (2 slices, 46 g)	0	11	4	85
Ham, cured, boneless, roasted (3 oz, 85 g)	0	20	8	151
Tenderloin, 1 raw chop with refuse, broiled (113 g)	0	23	6	153
Top loin (chops), boneless, 1 raw chop, broiled (113 g)	0	21	8	163
Poultry				
Chicken, drumsticks, battered and fried (43 g)	3	9	7	115
Chicken, wing meat, roasted (13 g)	0	4	1	26
Cornish game hens, meat and skin, roasted ($^1/_2$ bird, 129 g)	0	28	23	335
Cornish game hens, meat only, roasted ($^1/_2$ bird, 110 g)	0	25	4	147
Turkey, all classes, dark meat with skin, roasted (104 g)	0	28	12	230
Turkey, all classes, white meat with skin, roasted (112 g)	0	32	8	212
Vegetables				
Artichokes, boiled and drained, without salt ($^1/_2$ cup hearts, 84 g)	9	3	0	42
Asparagus, boiled and drained (4 spears, 60 g)	2	2	0	14
Beets, boiled and drained ($^1/_2$ cup slices, 85 g)	9	2	0	37
Broccoli, boiled and drained, without salt (1 medium stalk)	9	5	0	50
Broccoli raw (1 cup, 71 g)	4	2	0	20
Cabbage, boiled and drained, without salt ($^1/_2$ cup, 75 g)	3	1	0	17
Carrots, raw (1 cup, 110 g)	11	1	0	47
Cauliflower, boiled and drained, without salt (3 flowerets, 54 g)	2	1	0	12
Celery, raw (1 cup, 120 g)	5	1	0	19
Coleslaw (1 tablespoon)	1	0	0	6

Food Item	Carbs (g)	Protein (g)	Fat (g)	Calories
Corn, sweet, yellow, boiled, and drained, without salt (1 ear, 8 g)	2	0	0	9
Creamed corn, canned (1 cup, 256 g)	46	5	0	184
Cucumber, raw, peeled (1 cup, 119 g)	2	1	0	14
Eggplant, raw (1 cup, 82 g)	5	1	0	21
Garlic, raw (1 tsp, 3 g)	1	0	0	4
Ginger root, raw (1 tsp, 2 g)	0	0	0	1
Lentils, sprouted, stir-fried, without salt (100 g)	21	9	0	101
Lettuce, iceberg, raw (1 cup, 55 g)	1	1	0	7
Lettuce, romaine, raw (10 g)	0	0	0	1
Mushrooms, raw (1 cup, 70 g)	4	1	0	18
Onions, raw (1 cup, 115 g)	10	1	0	44
Parsley, raw (1 tbs, 4 g)	0	0	0	1
Peas, green, boiled and drained, without salt (1 cup, 160 g)	26	8	0	134
Peppers, hot chili, green, raw (1 pepper, 45 g)	4	1	0	18
Peppers, jalapeno, raw (1 pepper, 14 g)	1	0	0	4
Peppers, sweet green, raw (1 cup, 92 g)	6	1	0	25
Peppers, sweet yellow, raw (1 cup, 52 g)	3	1	0	14
Potatoes, baked, flesh, without salt ($\frac{1}{2}$ cup, 61 g)	13	1	0	57
Radishes, raw (1 large, 9 g)	0	0	0	2
Seaweed, kelp, raw (1/8 cup, 10 g)	1	0	0	4
Spinach, raw (1 cup, 56 g)	1	1	0	7
Squash, summer, raw (1 cup, 130 g)	5	1	0	25
Squash, winter, all varieties, raw (1 cup, 116 g)	10	1	0	43
Sweet potato, baked in skin, without salt (1 large, 180 g)	43	4	0	185
Tomatoes, green, raw (1 cup, 180 g)	9	2	0	43
Tomatoes, red, raw (1 cup, 149 g)	7	1	0	31
Tomatoes, sun-dried (1 piece, 2 g)	1	0	0	5
Yam, raw (1 cup, 150 g)	42	3	0	177

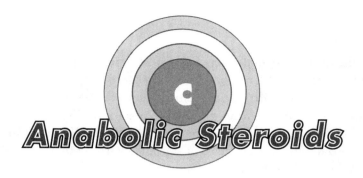

Anabolic Steroids

Anabolic: Promoting growth.

Steroid: A hormone with a cholesterol molecule. Sex hormones are steroids and contain anabolic factors. These derivatives of testosterone are synthesized from roots and are manmade copies of the male hormones released during and after puberty.

Anabolic steroids are known to help muscles grow by increasing the body's ability to retain protein. This increased availability of protein to muscle in turn increases its synthesis capabilities, thereby causing greater muscle mass and body weight.

Pharmaceutical steroids have been around for approximately fifty years now. It is believed that the first form of the drug was developed by scientists in Nazi Germany as a way to create a super race. At the end of World War II, this new technology was utilized to help restore life to American POWs. The Russians caught wind of this and enlisted some of their own captured German scientists to perfect the use of testosterone for their own athletes.

In the early fifties, the American scientist Dr. John Zeigler verified the use of testosterone in effectively improving the abilities of Russian weight lifters. He joined forces with CIBA laboratories to develop an enhancement drug for American athletes. Their research brought about Dianabol, a crude but effective derivative of testosterone, which is still in use today.

There are currently many designer steroids being developed all over the world. The newer drugs are modified testosterone derivatives, processed in a way to give you more of the growth factor. Unfortunately, they also deliver more of the side effects, or androgenic effects, that every steroid has. The androgenic effect enables you to perform sexually and develop body hair. On the downside, it also tends to cause acne, early maturity of bones, liver and prostate problems, water-weight gain due to salt retention, increasingly aggressive behavior, and shrunken testes; it can also stop the normal production of testosterone, which can lead to sterility.

The federal government and the Food and Drug Administration have verified the dangerous side effects of steroids, warning that using them can even kill you. On the other hand, pharmaceutical literature claims that anabolic steroids can prevent, or reverse, tissue depletion, as well as increase the retention and utilization of protein.

There is definitely a mixed message here because there are those who want to legalize steroids and have the medical industry regulate them. Wouldn't that just be jolly, considering that so many doctors are in the pocket of the drug companies. I can see it now—STUDIES SHOW REMARK-ABLE RESULTS FROM USING STEROIDS. And somewhere at the bottom the fine print would read: *Oh, by the way, using this drug may cause liver, kidney, and heart failure.*

Steroids belong nowhere in society except perhaps for use by those with anabolic problems, such as seniors, those with male menopause, and those recovering from injury or various diseases. But even under a doctor's supervision, caution must be used. Most physicians simply don't know the facts and are unaware of the long- and short-term effects of these drugs. The bottom line is that anabolic steroids are dangerous both physically and mentally.

No one more than myself, and perhaps a few dead bodybuilders and football players, can better describe the pitfalls and destructive power of anabolic steroids. Most champion bodybuilders and athletes are reluctant to discuss the horror stories connected to steroid use, which involve strokes, heart failure, artery disease, infertility, kidney and liver disorders, depression, and suicide, to name a few. "Riding high in April—Shot down in May" could be the theme for those who partake of these substances. I lost a couple of good friends to this stuff, and almost lost myself on more than one occasion.

It wasn't until I had won the Mr. America, and Mr. USA titles that I started this madness. Convinced against my better judgment, I joined the campaign of body destruction in order to compete in the Mr. Universe contest. It was obvious that the competitors at that level were bigger and harder than me, so I agreed to take steroids. I started out cautiously, taking one pill a day. When I started seeing the results, I began getting bolder and figured, if one pill works, two will work even better. Before you know it, you're taking a handful of anabolic steroids a day and injecting half a dozen shots a week. I actually believed nothing would happen to me. At the same time, there was no data as to the effect of this stuff, and after all, at that time doctors were giving it to us.

Slowly, I learned the harsh realities. At first, it was my mental state. I was more aggressive, meaner. You could say I was outright nasty. Then the headaches came. Headaches? They were more like jackhammers pounding at my brain. Oh, and yes, there were the nosebleeds. That was fun. All the while, I was getting bigger and bigger as my blood pressure rose higher and higher. Sure, I won the heavyweight division of the Mr. Universe competition all right, but at what price? To begin with, there was depression, impotency, and infertility. I was quite the man all right, a real Mr. Universe. I looked great, but the machinery didn't work. This went on for quite a while, until one day I woke up with this ghastly pain in my side. It was my body telling me, "Listen jerk, you're going to die if you don't quit this stuff." It turned out I had these tumorlike cysts the size of golf balls on my liver. Sometimes, life gets your ethics in even if you don't. This was one of those times. After that, I realized the absolute dangers that anabolic steroids pose to the body, and I stopped using steroids.

Fortunately, I healed up, and I have been on an anti-steroid campaign ever since. I have made it my business to promote the non-use of steroids and expose the dangers of these drugs. I've spent the greater part of my life researching alternative methods of producing muscles in order to provide a safe, healthy alternative to this deadly solution.

I tell this true story so others, particularly youthful athletes, can understand the dangers of these drugs and how destructive they can be. The unfortunate lure is that steroids work. They work well and they work fast.

There are those who try to claim that steroids don't enhance athletic ability or talent. Okay, what is talent? Talent is a measurement of the amount of ability you're willing to demonstrate at the present time. What? Yes, believe it or not, a lot of the time a human being is running on automatic, functioning on old pictures of events stored in the mind. Sports, however, more than any other event, requires a mind to operate in present time and be able to predict the future. For example, a golfer has to predict where the ground will curve and how that will affect the ball. A batter in baseball has to predict what the pitcher will throw and the pitcher needs to predict how the batter will swing. The only way a player can do this is if he's in present time communicating with the environment. A slump is basically a player out of present time. How he gets that way and gets back is another book.

In the past, not much attention was paid to the use of steroids. However, it was evident that they were being widely used by those like me. Today's headlines disclose the fact that many major athletes at the top of the athletic food chain have used steroids for years to achieve their goals. Society has become mechanical. There is very little free consciousness left. Hollywood, Madison Avenue, and some well-placed business concerns have shaped people's behavior. Acceptance by many has replaced the acceptance of self. There lies the problem. It is quite clear that the validation of others is the driving force behind the use of anabolic steroids, and drug abuse in general. The sheer fact that I am discussing this problem is a clear indication of the breakdown of the morals, ethics, and integrity of the families of these individuals. It is my belief that the entire problem stems from the lack of instilling in our young a sense of worth and self-respect—of integrity, and the ethic and moral values necessary to combat any aberrant viewpoint. Laws are passed because there is a breakdown in moral fiber. Government has to step in to handle what the individual can't.

I myself was a product of an abusive upbringing. I was suppressed, invalidated, and ignored. I would reach out and originate ideas and free thought only to be told to shut up, or punished for expressing a viewpoint. It is a funny thing about human beings—they crave acceptance and a sense of belonging and acknowledgment for who and what they are. If they are deprived of it at home, they will seek it elsewhere, via a gang or other outside groups. Thus, this new cult, gang, or muscle-building group will dictate the laws of behavior. The laws of bodybuilding are governed by the necessity to build a body at any cost. It becomes a solution to a problem of acceptance and validation. So don't blame steroids or any other body-enhancing drugs. They are only the byproduct of a fallen society and a failed family unit. In my travels around the country and around the world, I have observed individuals as young as eleven or twelve years old starting out with some form of anabolic steroids to increase their athletic ability or appearance. So, since the 1980s, I have made it my goal to rid the world of these dangerous drugs. I've attended many seminars on this topic. What I've learned through my spiritual and mind training was that, in order to handle any kind of problem, you must have a solution to that problem. The current solution chosen by the so-called learned people in this field is to try to scare people out of using steroids. Well, everyone knows this absolutely does not work. It hasn't worked with other drugs, such as alcohol, cocaine, or heroin; and fear certainly hasn't worked in the criminal system either, where perpetrators are threatened with jail and the death penalty.

All addiction starts out as a solution to a problem. You will never solve addiction—never. What you can solve is the problem that leads to the addiction. Usually, this addiction stems from some inability to confront life on some level. It is a solution to some fear that cannot be solved.

The unfortunate truth is, once an individual has chosen the steroid solution, it is extremely difficult to convince her or him to come off steroids. I believe you must address those who are thinking about using them *before* they do. It's my belief that, if you can present enough evidence in a strong and reality-breaking manner to expose the real dangers connected to their use, while offering an alternative solution, you may have a chance. Otherwise, life will have to deliver their ethics with some unfortunate illnesses, as it did to me.

The desire to be strong and look good is not an addiction; it is a natural desire. It stems from an innate purpose, to duplicate what occurs in nature, which is to survive and create. A person's need to be competitive, to be better, stronger, faster, and smarter than the next person can be traced back to our earliest ancestors. These qualities amounted to survival during cavedwelling times and they remain so in civilized society today. Steroids effectively enhance these coveted qualities, but they unfortunately create this effect by mutating the body into a state it would not normally have reached.

High testosterone levels were necessary to early existence. When humans first appeared on earth, they were like any other animals, guided by instinct, urges, and compulsions. High-steroid levels increased early man's aggression and sex drive. Barbaric behavior was a survival tool. Strength and speed were early man's only weapons against a vengeful planet, while procreation and survival of the group depended on an uncontrolled sexual urge. Early man was programmed and guided by his genes, which allowed the body to produce massive amounts of steroids and hormones to assure his continued existence.

Today, however, people live under a different set of rules and laws, in a society where hostile behavior and sexual aggression cannot be tolerated. When an individual takes steroids, a lot of the animal instincts clearly manifest themselves again. It's as if the body is being programmed to deal with a dangerous non-survival environment again. The urges are overwhelming and the sexual appetite cannot be satisfied. Spirituality, ethics, integrity, and a sense of what is right and wrong are often replaced by the needs, desires, and urges associated with the animal kingdom. Although this method of survival may have been effective thousands of years ago, it is certainly not a desirable condition today. The steroid solution to the problem of survival of the fittest is far from ideal. It is ultimately harmful, not only to the individual, but to society as well.

I have made it my life's work to find a solution to the steroid problem. What will build muscle and strength and athletic ability without anabolic steroids? I believe Atomic Fitness, my method of Intensity/Insanity, is that solution. I've seen how it has worked and does work. So my pursuit now is to create a situation where, by learning the proper ways of exercising and eating, and the proper philosophy of the mind, a young man or young woman will be able to overcome all barriers and do it in a natural and healthy way. My findings are extraordinary, and as you come to understand the concepts I have outlined, you'll know this to be true.

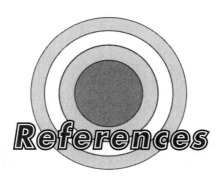

References

BOOKS

Darwin, Charles. *Origin of the Species.* New York, NY: New American Library, 2003.

Hatfield, Frederick. *Fitness, The Complete Guide.* New York, NY: McGraw-Hill, 1994.

Hubbard, L. Ron. *Dianetics: The Modern Science of Mental Health.* Los Angeles, CA: Bridge Publications, Reissue edition, May 1995.

Hubbard, L. Ron. *The Science of Survival.* Reissue edition. Los Angeles, CA: Bridge Publications, 2005.

Hubbard, L. Ron. *Technical Dictionary.* Los Angeles, CA: Bridge Publications, Reprint Edition, 1987.

Pearl, Bill. *Keys to the Inner Universe.* Reprint edition. Phoenix, OR: Bill Pearl Enterprises, 2000.

Wolcott, William. *The Metabolic Typing Diet.* New York, NY: Broadway Books, 2000.

NEWSLETTERS

Arnold, Dara. *Better Health for Better Living.* Baltimore, MD: Healthier News, Institute for Cooperative Medicine, 2005.

Holford, Patrick. *The Wellness Advisor: Optimum Health & Natural Healing.* Potomac, MD: Patrick Holford's Wellness Advisor, 2005.

Marchione, Victor. *The Food Doctor.* Boston, MA: Doctor's Health Press, 2005.

"Nature's Miracle Worker." Special Research Report. Hueytown, AL: Health Resources, 2005.

Rowens, Robert Jay. *Second Opinion*. Atlanta, GA: Second Opinion Publishing, 2005.

Sinatra, Dr. Stephen. *Heart, Health and Nutrition: A Cardiologist's Guide to Total Wellness*. Potomac, MD: Healthy Directions, 2005.

Swartzberg, John. "Is it Wise to be a Weekend Warrior?" Berkeley, CA: *U.C. Berkeley Wellness Letter*, September 2005.

Thompson, Jenny. *The Health Sciences Institute*. Baltimore, MD: Institute for Health Sciences, January 2005.

Weil, Andrew. *Self Healing, Creating Optimum Health for Your Body and Soul*. Watertown, MA: Body and Soul Omnimedia, Inc., May 2005.

Whitaker, Julian. *Health and Healing*. Potomac, MD: Healthy Directions, January 27, 2005.

Williams, David G. *Alternatives for the Health Conscious Individual*. Potomac, MD: Mountain Home Publishing, January 2005.

West, Bruce. *Health Alert*. Hotchkiss, CO: Health Alert/Immune Systems, Inc., October 2004.

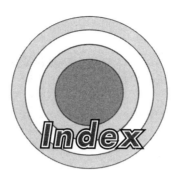

Index

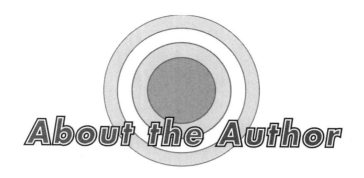

About the Author

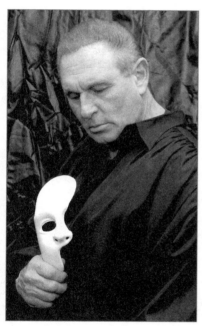

Steve Michalik, a triple-crown body building champion known as "The Phantom," whose titles include Mr. USA, Mr. America, and Mr. Universe, among twenty-two various other titles, began developing his Atomic Fitness System of training as a youth. Steve's philosophy of mind over body, in combination with his principles of Atomic Fitness—compressing time, space, and energy to increase matter—enabled him to achieve tremendous successes and conquer enormous physical and mental barriers throughout his life. Today, Steve teaches Atomic Fitness to time-strapped homemakers and corporate leaders alike. His clients are constantly amazed at their ability to transform their physiques in a fraction of the time they were previously investing.

Steve is also active in the campaign against steroids. He is constantly sought after to offer his experience and expertise on the dangers of steroid abuse, and he leads a team of natural bodybuilders who consistently dominate the stage. To this day, Steve remains dedicated to maintaining physical and mental well-being. He never misses a workout and is a constant source of inspiration to those he mentors.